Atlas of Endoscopic Plastic Surgery

Edoardo Raposio
Editor

Atlas of Endoscopic Plastic Surgery

Springer

Editor
Edoardo Raposio
University of Parma
Parma
Italy

ISBN 978-3-319-19460-8 ISBN 978-3-319-19461-5 (eBook)
DOI 10.1007/978-3-319-19461-5

Library of Congress Control Number: 2015949933

Springer Cham Heidelberg New York Dordrecht London

Printed on acid-free paper

Springer International Publishing AG Switzerland is part of Springer Science+Business Media (www.springer.com)

To my sons Jacopo and Giorgio Gualtiero

Preface

The adage "large incision, big surgeon" governed surgery for over 100 years. The larger the wound, however, the more skin, fascia, nerves, and muscles are transected, and the more morbidity can be expected.

Surgeons from various domains have become fascinated by endoscopy, with its very low complication rates, high diagnostic yields, and the possibility of performing a large variety of therapeutic procedures. During the past 30 years, the number and diversity of endoscopic surgical procedures has advanced rapidly, with many new methods for both diagnosis and treatment.

Since the breakthrough of endoscopic surgical procedures in medicine at the end of the 1980s, there has been an enormous evolution in endoscopic surgery, not only in general surgery but also in plastic surgery. Concomitantly, the equipment, endoscopes, and instruments also have evolved greatly. The main intention of this book is to give surgeons a reference to consult when they want to embark on endoscopic plastic surgical procedures that they have not carried out before. Indeed, this atlas is an educational resource not only for plastic surgeons in training but also for those well established in practice.

The book concentrates on explanations of techniques that are illustrated in detail. Experts from all over the world have contributed to the book. This first edition of *Endoscopic Plastic Surgery Atlas* provides detailed, step-by-step instructions on how to perform state-of-the-art endoscopic surgical techniques in the complex field of plastic surgery. More than 300 high-quality photographs help to clarify complex techniques throughout the book.

There is consensus that endoscopic surgery is more difficult than open surgery: the view is two-dimensional, the entrance ports are fixed, and the tips of the instruments have only a very limited number of degrees of freedom of movement. No wonder that most endoscopic surgical procedures take longer and are more fatiguing for the surgeon. The question "Is it worth the trouble?" must be answered. Worth considering are the many advantages of endoscopic procedures: smaller incisions and less tissue trauma, improved illumination and visibility, reduced blood loss, less postoperative pain, earlier mobilization, lower overall morbidity, easier operative approach in obese patients, earlier return to work and activities, lower complication rates, easier revision surgery because of less scar tissue, greater possibility of outpatient procedures, less need for postoperative pain medication, and lower costs due to shorter inpatient stays.

Endoscopic Plastic Surgery Atlas represents a comprehensive description of the current endoscopic techniques in reconstructive and aesthetic plastic surgery. It supplies surgeons with all the information necessary to successfully accomplish an endoscopic approach to various plastic surgery procedures, from carpal and cubital tunnel release to breast augmentation and reconstruction, from migraine surgery to hyperhidrosis management, from facial aesthetic surgery to flap and fascia lata harvesting, from mastectomy to abdominal wall surgery.

Parma, Italy — Edoardo Raposio

Acknowledgments

I want to thank all the contributing authors for giving their precious time to write their chapters and share their great experiences:

Daniel M. Avery III, MD (USA)
Miles G. Berry, MD, MS, FRCS (UK)
Nicholas M. Caggiano, MD (USA)
Giorgia Caruana, MD (Italy)
Nicholas A. Flugstad, MD (USA)
Joseph P. Hunstad, MD (USA)
Yoko Katsuragi-Tomioka, MD (Japan)
Ai Koyanagi, MD, PhD (Spain)
Kristofer S. Matullo, MD (USA)
Stephen Morley, MD, FRCS (UK)
Masahiro Nakagawa, MD (Japan)
Paul M. Rea, MBChB, MSc, PhD (UK)
Manash Ranjan Sahoo, MD (India)
José Maria Serra-Mestre, MD (Italy)
José Maria Serra-Renom, MD (Spain)
Jan J. Stanek, MD, FRCS (UK)
Nobuyuki Takemoto, MD, PhD (Japan)
Hiroshi Yamamoto, MD, PhD (Japan)
Hisamitsu Zaha, MD (Japan)

Contents

Contributors

Daniel M. Avery III, MD Department of Orthopaedic Surgery, St. Luke's University Hospital, Bethlehem, PA, USA

Miles G. Berry, MS, FRCS (Plast) Surgical Aesthetics, London, England, UK

Nicholas M. Caggiano, MD Department of Orthopedic Surgery, St. Luke's University Hospital, Bethlehem, PA, USA

Giorgia Caruana, MD Department of Surgical Science, Plastic Surgery Department, Parma University Hospital, Parma, Italy

Nicholas A. Flugstad, MD The Hunstad Kortesis Center for Cosmetic Plastic Surgery, Huntersville, NC, USA

Joseph P. Hunstad, MD, FACS The Hunstad Kortesis Center for Cosmetic Plastic Surgery, Huntersville, NC, USA

Division of Plastic Surgery, The University of North Carolina, Chapel Hill, NC, USA

Plastic Surgery Division, Department of Surgery, Carolinas Medical Ctr., University Hospital, Charlotte, NC, USA

Yoko Katsuragi-Tomioka, MD Division of Plastic and Reconstructive Surgery, Shizuoka Cancer Center Hospital, Naga-izumi, Shizuoka, Japan

Ai Koyanagi, MD, MSc, PhD Research and Development Unit, Parc Sanitari Sant Joan de Déu, Fundació Sant Joan de Déu, Dr. Antoni Pujadas, Barcelona, Spain

Kristofer S. Matullo, MD Department of Orthopedic Surgery, St. Luke's University Hospital and Health Network, Bethlehem, PA, USA

Stephen Morley, MD, FRCS (Plast) Canniesburn Plastic Surgery Unit, Glasgow Royal Infirmary, Glasgow, UK

Masahiro Nakagawa, MD, PhD Division of Plastic and Reconstructive Surgery, Shizuoka Cancer Center Hospital, Naga-izumi, Shizuoka, Japan

Edoardo Raposio, MD, PhD, FICS Plastic Surgery Section, Department of Surgical Sciences, University of Parma, Italy, Parma, Italy

Paul M. Rea, MBChB, MSc, DipFMS, FHEA, PhD, MIMI, RMIP, FRSA Laboratory of Human Anatomy, Room 349, School of Life Sciences, College of Medical, Veterinary, and Life Sciences, University of Glasgow, Glasgow, UK

Manash Ranjan Sahoo, MS, FAIS, FMAS, FALS Department of Surgery, Sriram Chandra Bhanj Medical College, Cuttack, Odisha, India

José Maria Serra-Mestre, MD Institute of Aesthetic and Plastic Surgery Dr. Serra Renom, Hospital Quiron, Barcelona Universitat, Internacional de Catalunya, Barcelona, Spain

José Maria Serra-Renom, MD, PhD Institute of Aesthetic and Plastic Surgery Dr. Serra Renom, Hospital Quiron, Barcelona Universitat, Internacional de Catalunya, Barcelona, Spain

Jan J. Stanek, MA, FRCS Surgical Aesthetics, London, UK

Nobuyuki Takemoto, MD, PhD Department of Breast and Endocrine Surgery, Japan Medical Alliance, Higashi Saitama General Hospital, Satte, Saitama, Japan

Hiroshi Yamamoto, MD, PhD Geriatric Health Service Facility, Yokohama Brain and Spine Center, Japan Medical Alliance, Yokohama, Kanagawa, Japan

Hisamitsu Zaha, MD Department of Breast Surgery, Nakagami Hospital, Okinawa-City, Okinawa, Japan

1 Endoscope-Assisted Brow Lift

Jan J. Stanek and Miles G. Berry

The brow-periorbita is a watershed region with a foot in two anatomical camps: The brow formally demarcates the limit of the face's upper third, but the eyes are technically part of the middle third. Obviously the two are anatomically and functionally inseparable, a point emphasised recently by the appellation *brow-lid continuum* [1]. Moreover, the brow has been described as both more resistant to senescence than the mid and lower face [2], yet prone to premature aging [3] by reason of the periorbita's more delicate skin and minimal subcutaneous padding. This conundrum may well be explained by regional anatomical differences: The thicker-skinned medial brow is actively supported by the frontalis, whereas the thinner lateral aspect lacks both intrinsic support and an antigravity muscle.

The evolution of brow lifting since its origin in 1919 has been well charted. Four key phases can be delineated (Table 1.1). The first lasted almost 40 years and was characterised by some form of direct excision [4–7]. The latter part of this time saw a decline in popularity because of poor longevity, a feature shared with the skin-only facelifts of the time. A paradigm shift ushered in the second era of muscle modification, either directly [8–10] or indirectly through denervation [11]. The third phase was typified by comprehending the importance of adequate ligamentous release [12–14]. The fourth and current era introduced the endoscope to plastic surgery [15, 16]. The improved vascularity of the endoscopically elevated forehead flap has further widened its application by permitting synchronous treatments such as CO_2 laser resurfacing [17].

Table 1.1 Key landmarks in the evolution of surgical brow rejuvenation

Phase	Year	Author	Key contribution
Phase I: "excision"	1919	Passot [4]	First description of surgical brow elevation through various excisions, including temporal
	1926	Hunt [5]	Coronal incisions both within and at anterior hairline
	1930	Passot [6]	Direct superciliary incision with undermining and elliptical excision
	1939	Fomon [7]	Forehead undermining and transection of pericranium
Phase II: "muscle"	1957	Bames [8]	Cross-hatching of frontalis to reduce its activity
	1957	Edwards [11]	Frontal branch transection to address frontalis hyperactivity
	1964	Marino and Gandolfo [10]	Modification of frontalis and corrugator supercilii
	1977	Kaye [9]	Frontalis and corrugator resection
Phase III: "release"	1976	Viñas et al. [12]	Elevation without tension via wide periorbital dissection and transverse galea-frontalis stripectomy
	1979	Pitanguy [13]	Multiple transverse and vertical galeal releases in glabella region
	1982	Owsley [14]	Comprehensive superior orbital rim release for durability
Phase IV: "endoscopic"	1992	Vasconez [15]	Initial presentation
	1994	Isse [16]	First publication
	1997	Ramirez and Pozner [17]	Synchronous CO_2 laser resurfacing

J.J. Stanek, MA, FRCS • M.G. Berry, MS, FRCS (Plast) (✉)
Surgical Aesthetics, 60 Wimpole Street, London W1G 8AG, UK
e-mail: mail@janstanek.com; info@milesgberry.com

E. Raposio (ed.), *Atlas of Endoscopic Plastic Surgery*, DOI 10.1007/978-3-319-19461-5_1

1.1 Surgical Procedure

1.1.1 Preparation and Equipment

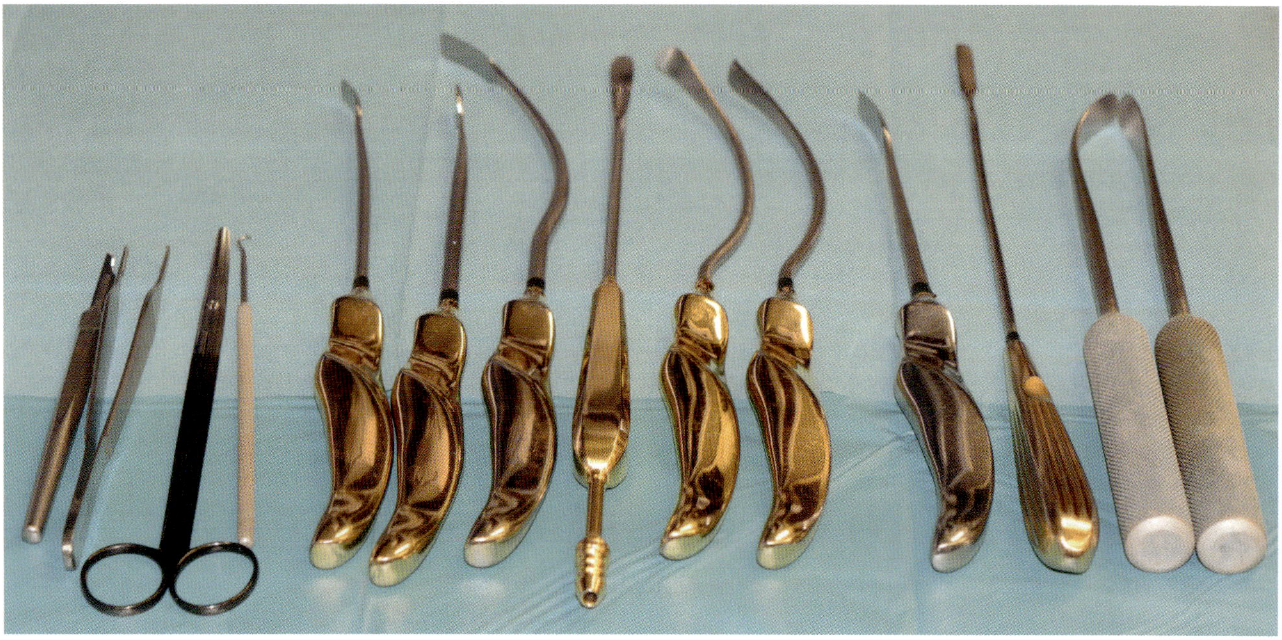

Fig. 1.1 A standard set of equipment for endoscopic brow lift

1.1.2 Markings

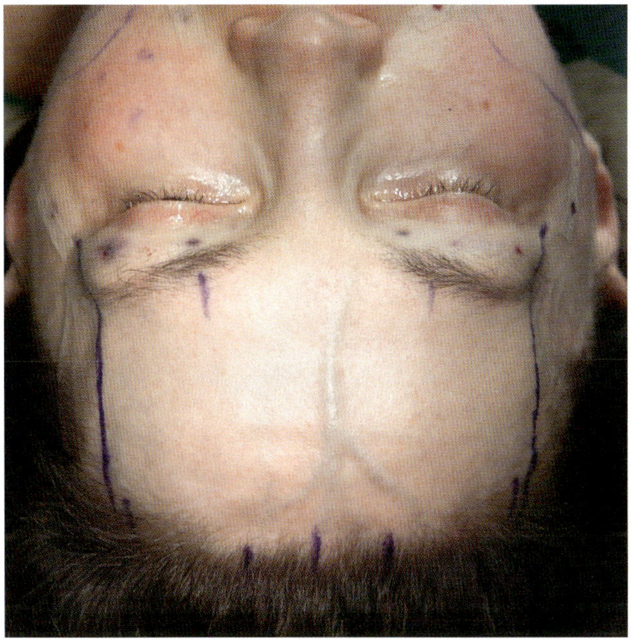

Fig. 1.2 Key markings showing the temporal line of fusion with central and paramedian access ports at the hairline

1.1.3 Infiltration

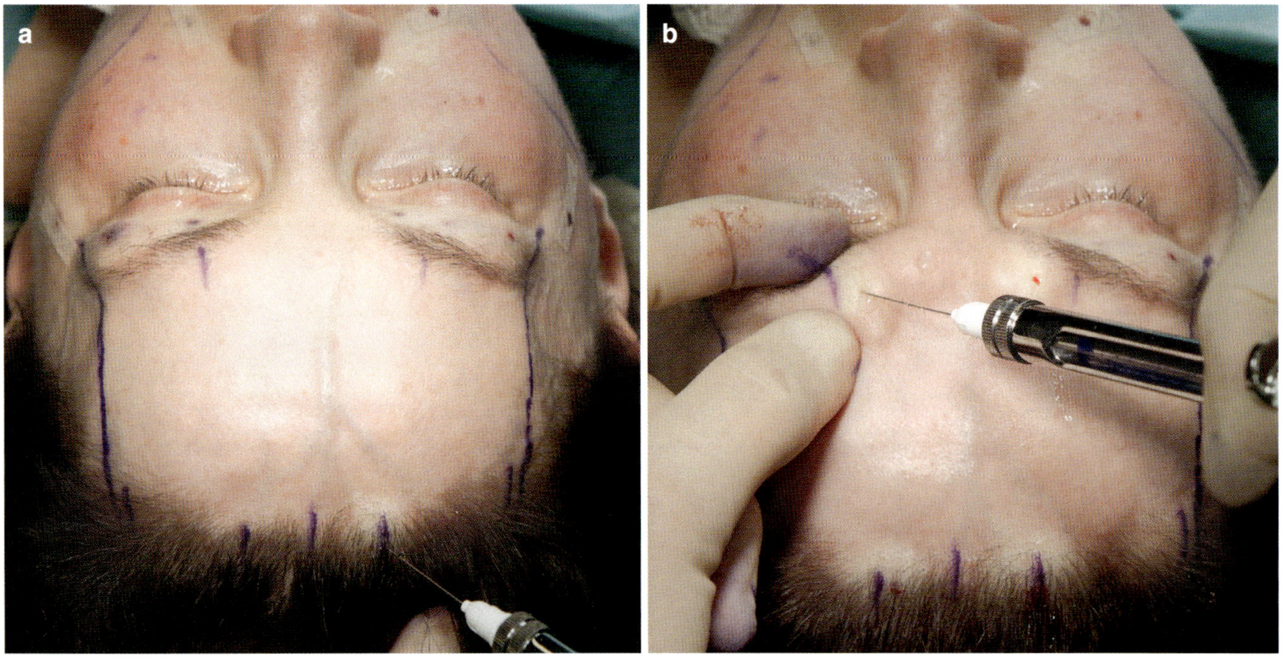

Fig. 1.3 Infiltration of 2 % lignocaine with 1-in-80,0000 adrenaline for the incisions (**a**) and muscle (**b**)

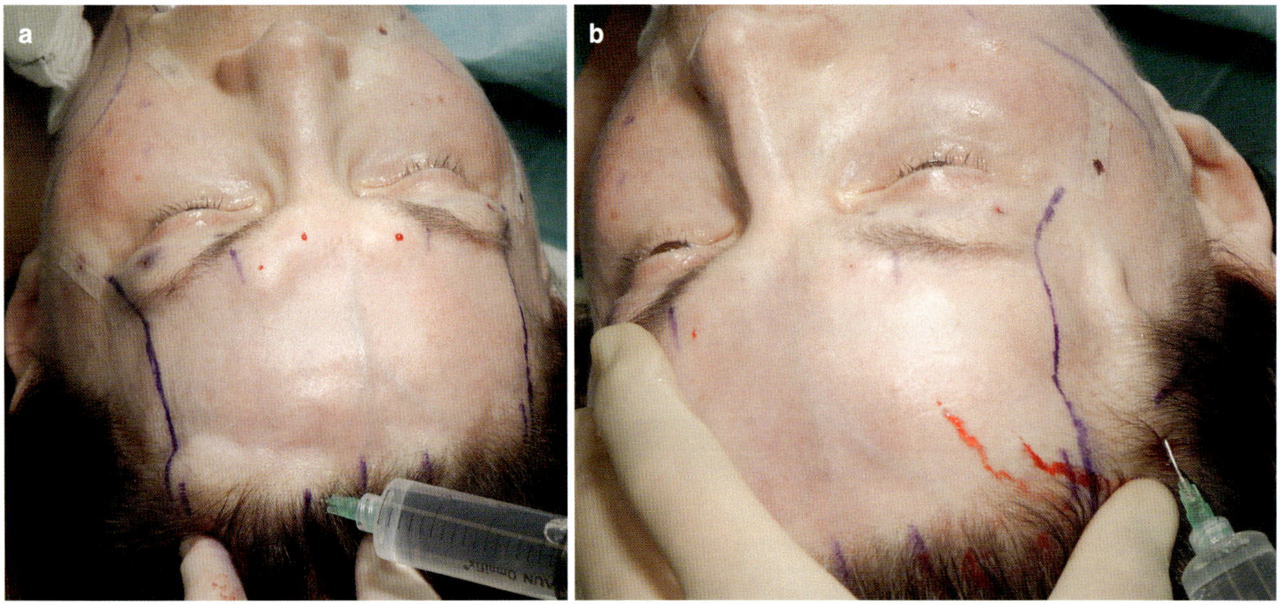

Fig. 1.4 Infiltration with a more dilute solution in the subperiosteal (**a**) and subtemporalis (**b**) planes to commence hydrodissection

1.1.4 Incision and Initial Dissection of the Central Pocket

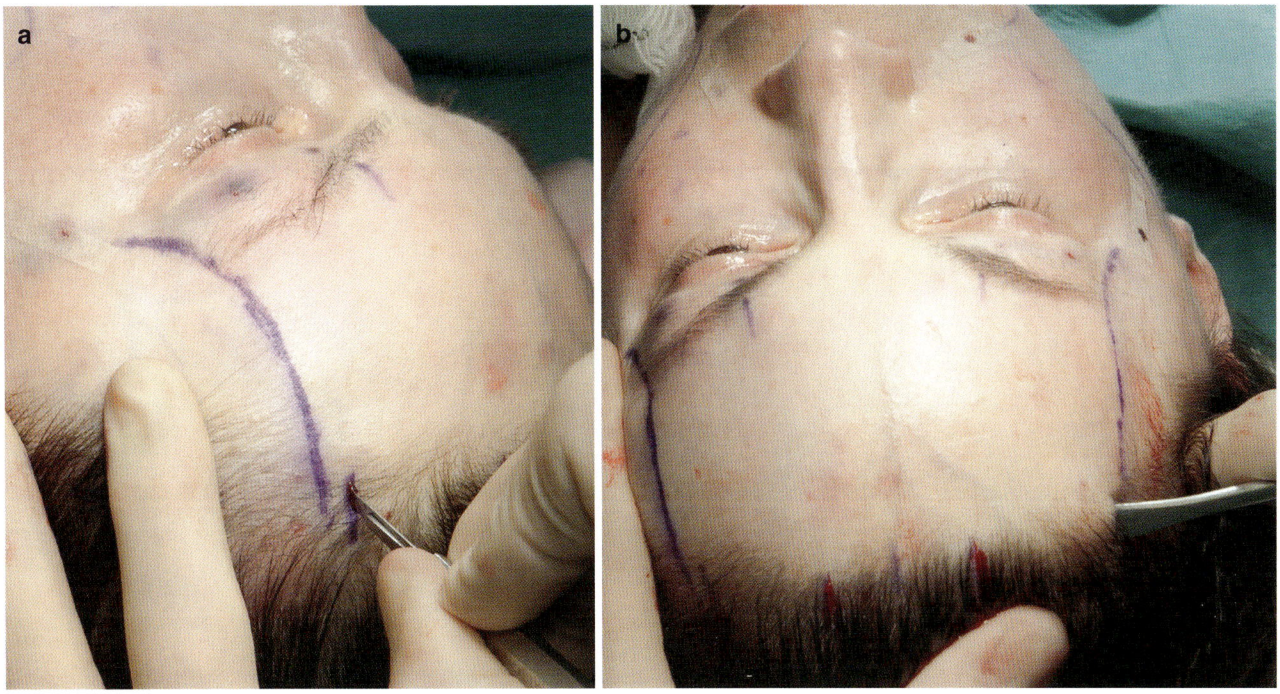

Fig. 1.5 Incision is perpendicular to the skin and direct to the bone (**a**), followed by limited posterior subperiosteal dissection (**b**). This dissection is usually no more than 1–2 cm behind the hairline, depending on the forehead height and how much elevation is required

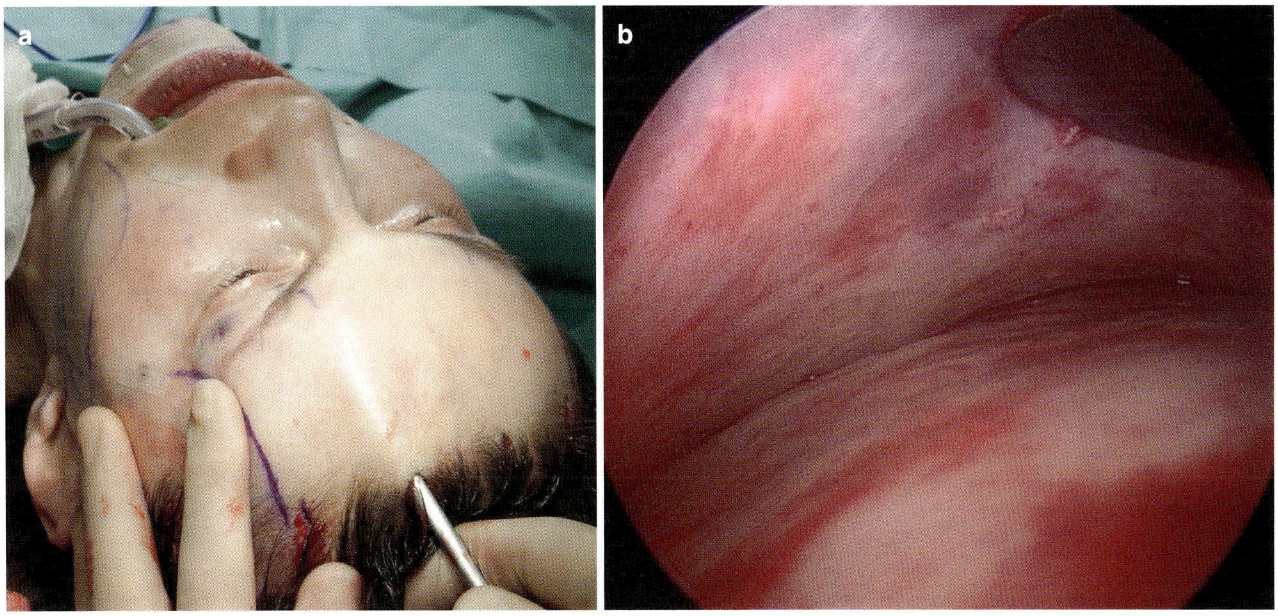

Fig. 1.6 Subperiosteal central compartment dissection is performed blind, laterally to the temporal lines of fusion (TLF) (**a**) and inferiorly to 2 cm above the brow (**b**)

1.1.5 Incision and Initial Dissection of the Temporal Pocket

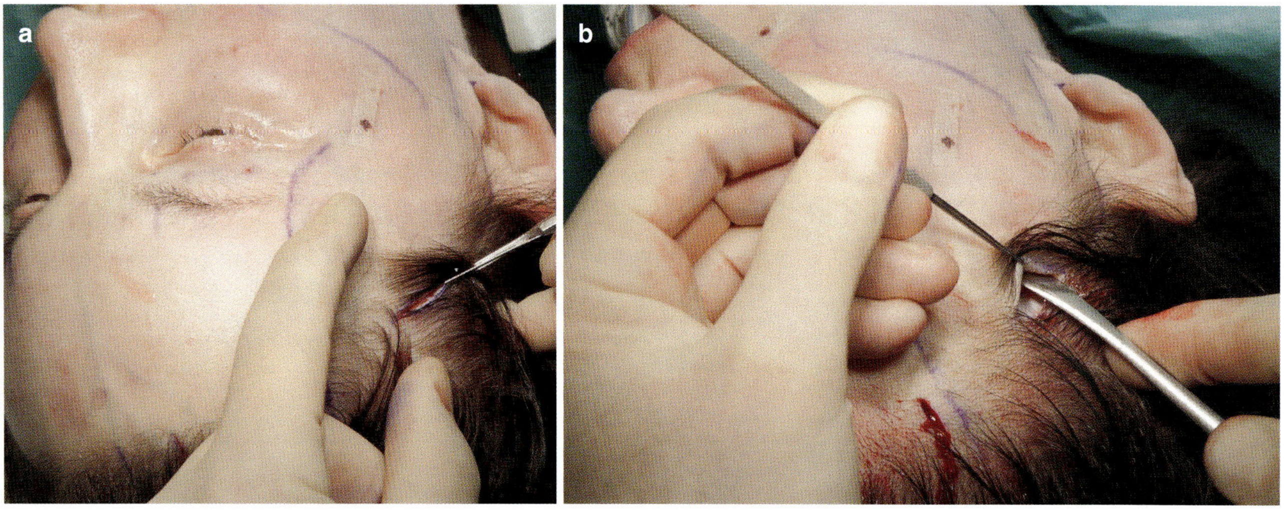

Fig. 1.7 The temporal incision is longer (2 cm) and runs perpendicular to a line subtended from the alar base through the lateral canthus (**a**). Temporal pocket dissection is also performed blind, but occurs on the glistening white, superficial surface of the deep temporal fascia (**b**)

1.1.6 Connection of Pockets, Temporal Lines of Fusion, and Sentinel Vein

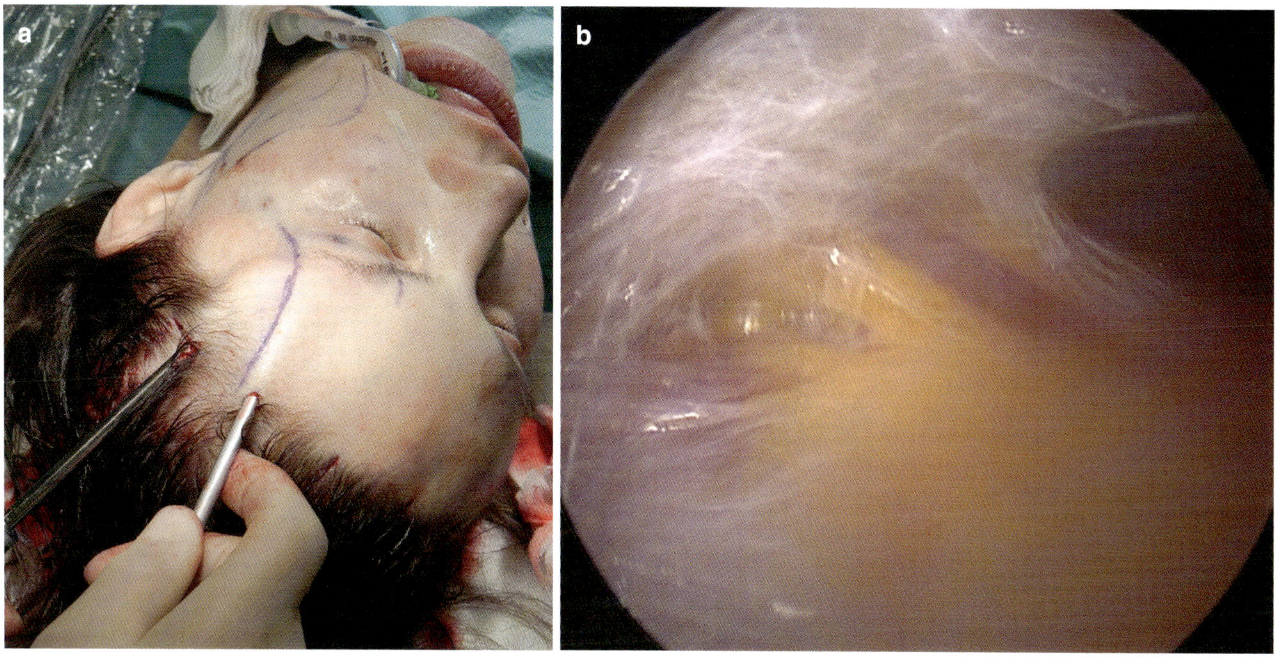

Fig. 1.8 The central and temporal compartments are then connected under direct vision (**a**). The "sentinel" vein (**b**) is clearly seen in the lateral fat pad and is the marker for the frontal branch of the facial nerve, which courses immediately lateral

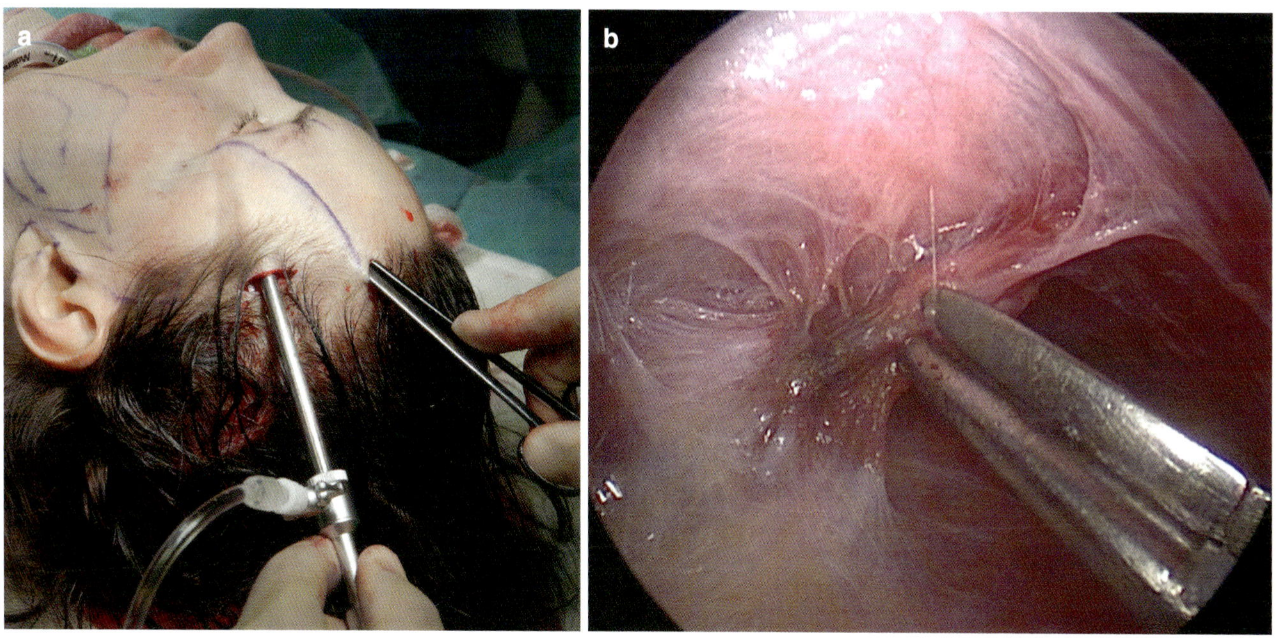

Fig. 1.9 The central and temporal compartments are then connected (**a**) by dividing the temporal line of fusion (**b**)

1.1.7 Inferior Periosteal Division and Open Muscle Disruption

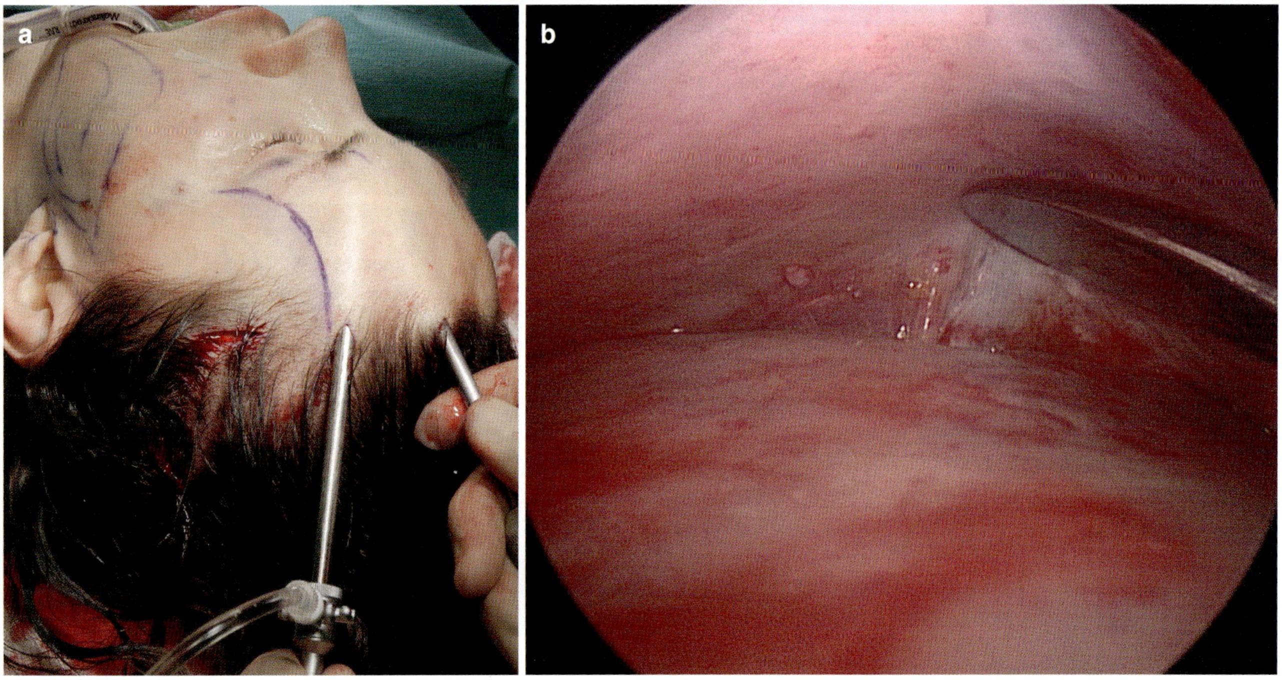

Fig. 1.10 Controlled subperiosteal dissection (**a**) yields a clean cavity, which allows for ready identification of the supraorbital neurovascular bundle. Usually exiting from its own foramen, it is generally the first neurovascular bundle to be encountered with a subperiosteal dissection (**b**)

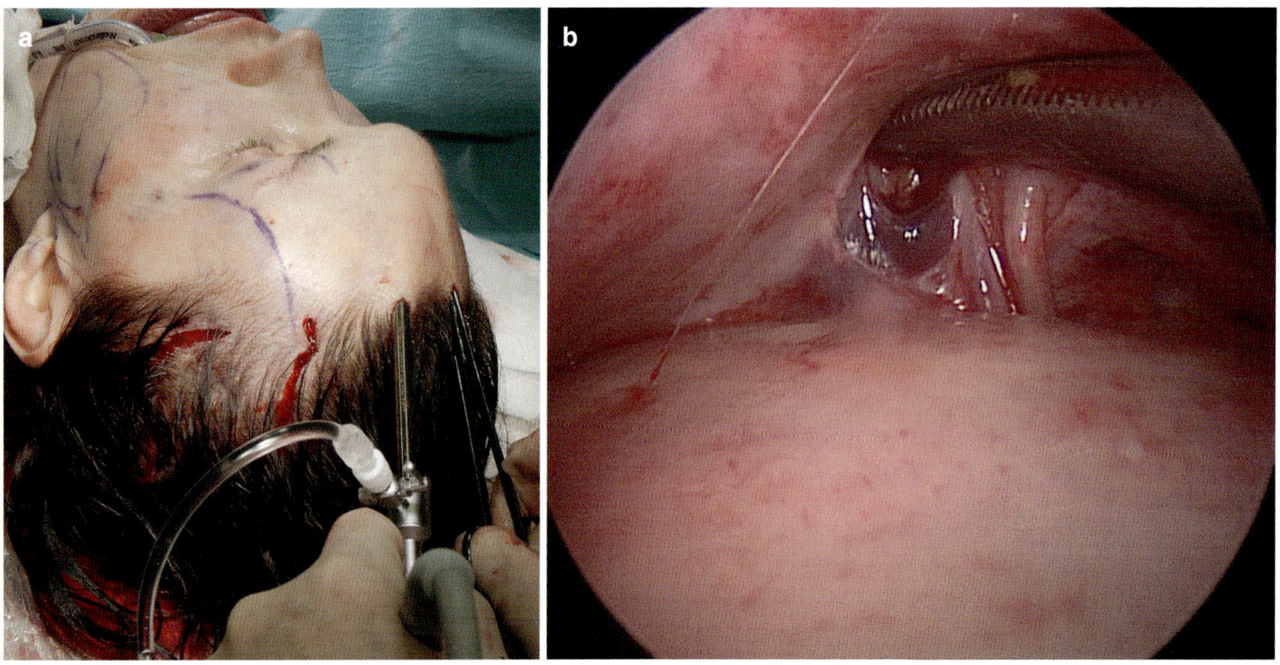

Fig. 1.11 Once through the paramedian periosteum, the supratrochlear neurovascular structures may be sought (**a**). Gentle muscle disruption should be used, rather than incision (**b**), as these structures sit within the bulk of the corrugator muscle

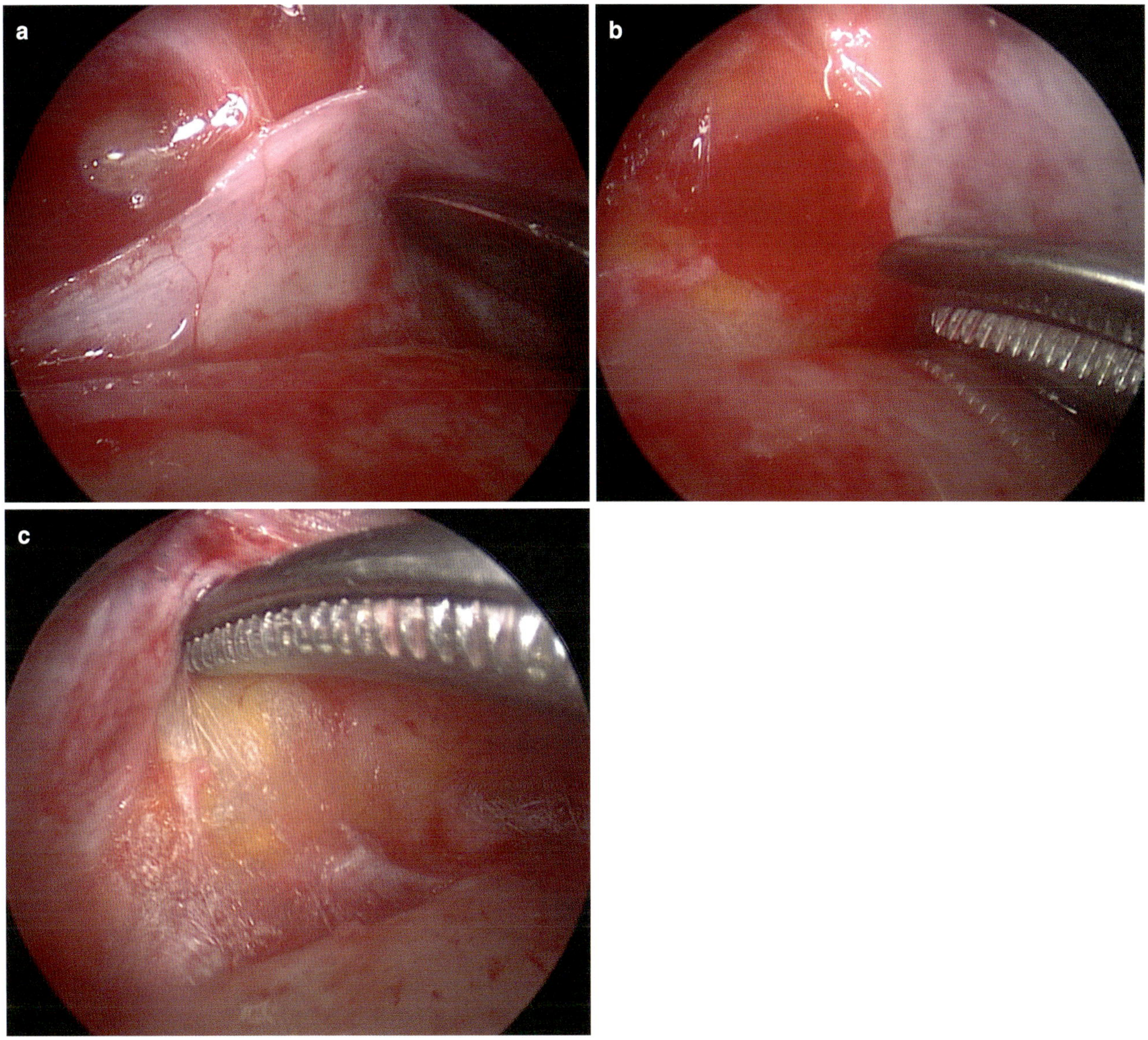

Fig. 1.12 When these important structures have been identified and preserved, the periosteum can then be released (**a**, **b**), as shown here by the periocular fat (**c**) as it sits within the bulk of the corrugator muscle

1.1.8 Closure and Fixation

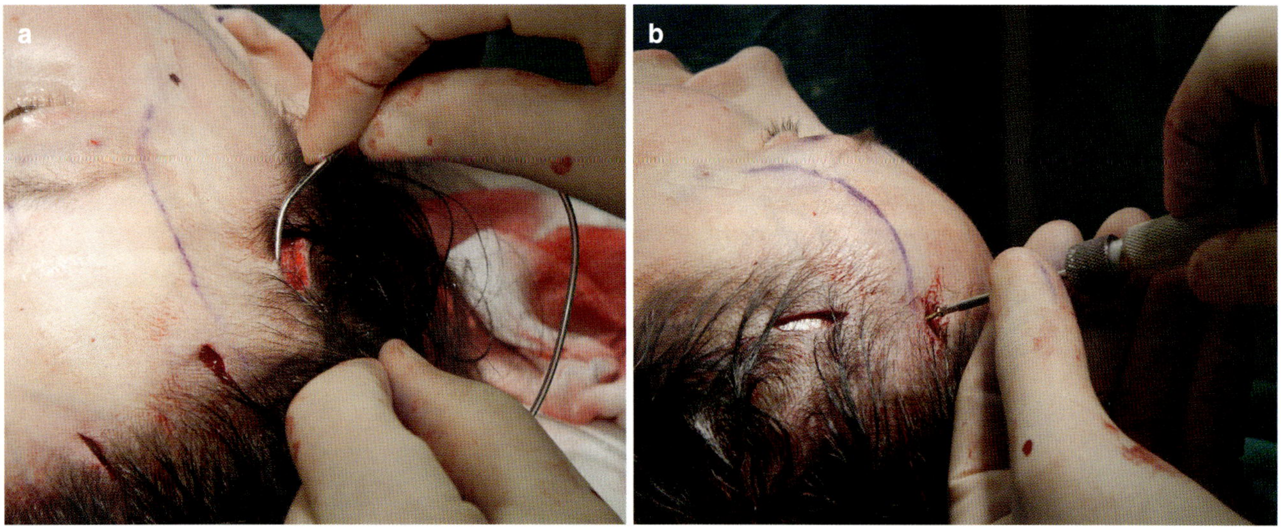

Fig. 1.13 An 8 Ch concertina drain is inserted into each side and brought out through the hair (**a**). Cortical screws (1.6×10–12 mm) have stood the test of time and are gently inserted into the outer table of the cranium, leaving only 2–3 mm protruding (**b**)

1.1.9 Elevation

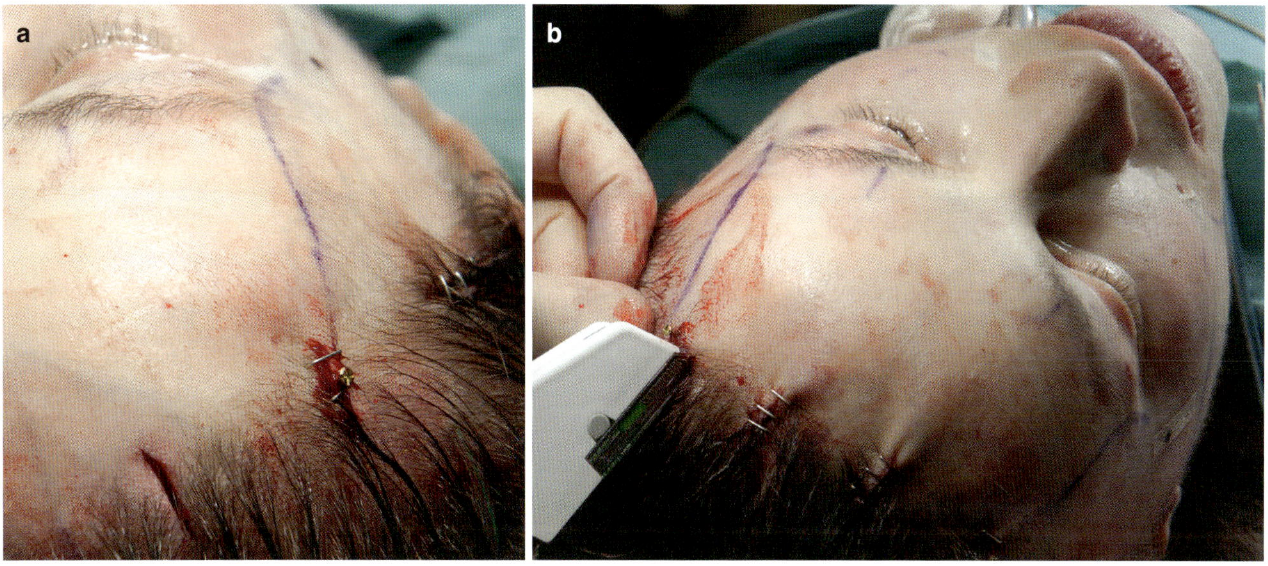

Fig. 1.14 The degree of brow "lift" is determined by traction on the skin and anchoring behind the screws with skin staples (**a**). The remaining forehead incisions are closed similarly (**b**)

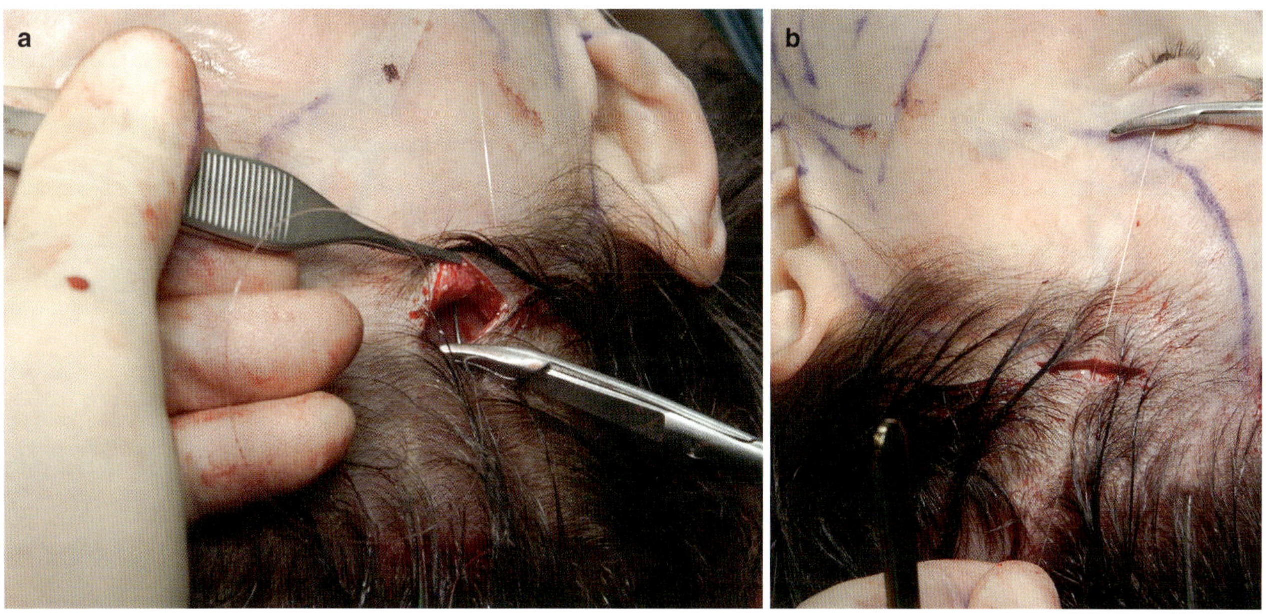

Fig. 1.15 A degree of temporal lift is provided, if required, by suturing anteriorly placed superficial temporal fascia (STF) (**a**) onto posteriorly sited deep temporal fascia (DTF) (**b**)

1.2 Clinical Examples

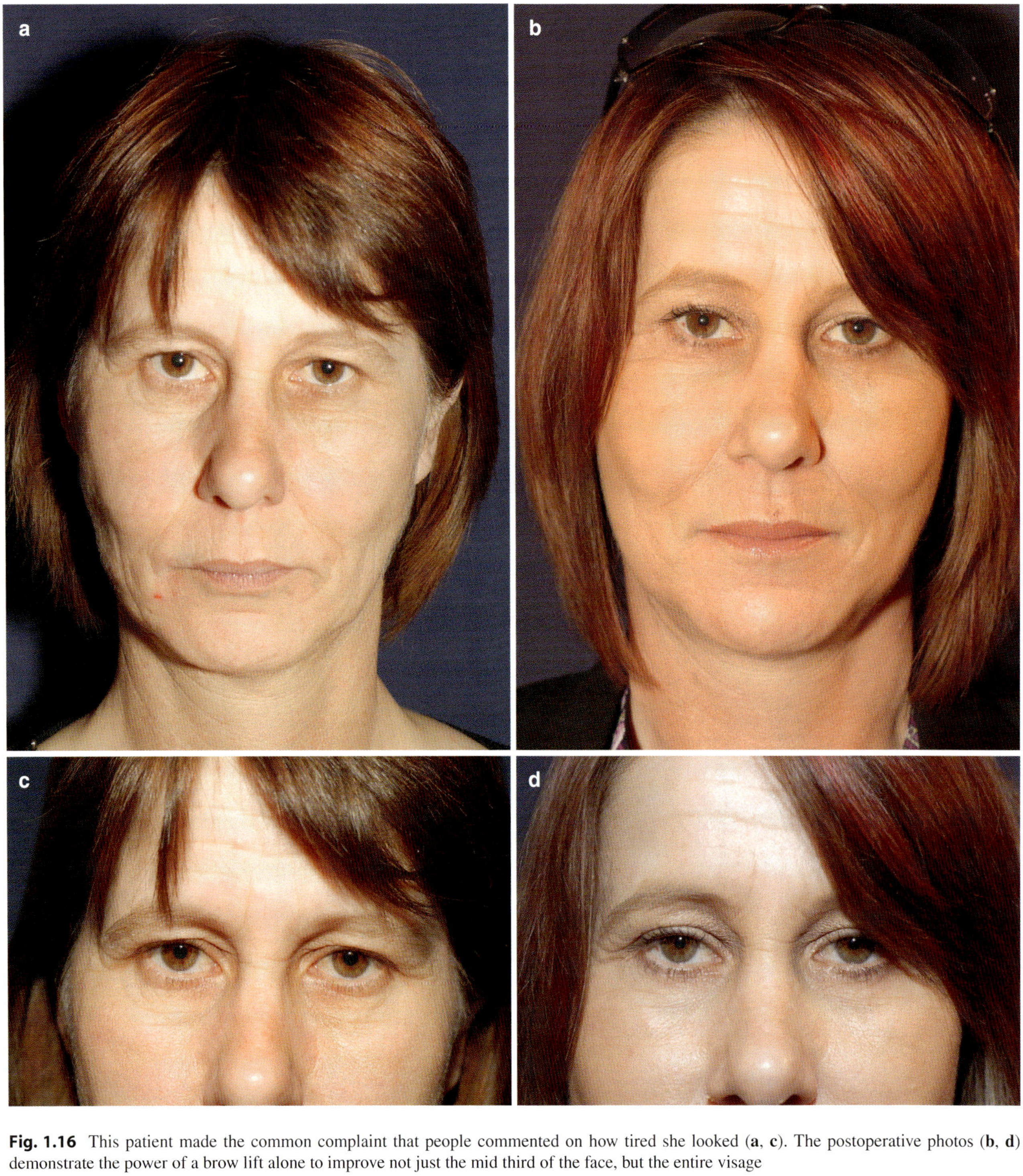

Fig. 1.16 This patient made the common complaint that people commented on how tired she looked (**a**, **c**). The postoperative photos (**b**, **d**) demonstrate the power of a brow lift alone to improve not just the mid third of the face, but the entire visage

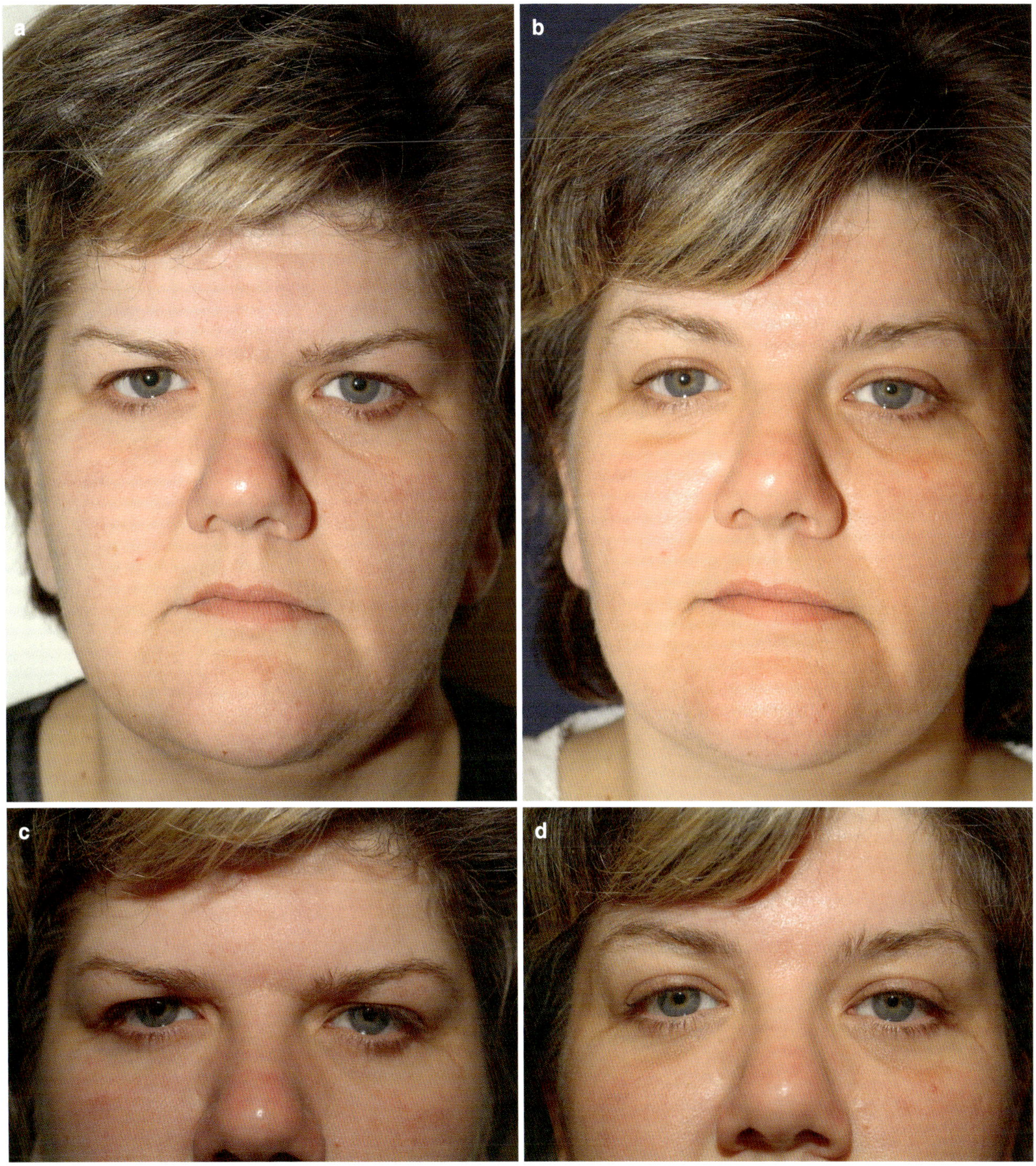

Fig. 1.17 Another use of the brow lift is demonstrated on this patient, whose congenitally low brow portrayed an angry appearance (**a**, **c**). In the postoperative photos (**b**, **d**), the brows have been elevated, their shape improved, and the apparent dermatochalasis managed without the need for upper blepharoplasty

1.3 Conclusions

1.3.1 Philosophy

Endoscopic brow lift is now well established and is a reliable and repeatable technique provided certain fundamental principles are followed:

- Creation of three optical cavities (two temporal and one frontal)
- Controlled posterior subperiosteal dissection
- Arcus marginalis and lateral orbital ligamentous attachment release as far as the lateral canthus, to enable cephalad brow repositioning
- Variable attenuation of glabellar complex muscles proportionate to their degree of hyperactivity
- Fixation performed routinely with temporary cortical screws. More marked asymmetry can be approached with the Endotine device (MicroAire, Charlottesville, VA, USA) or cortical bone tunnels

1.3.2 Indications

Endoscopic brow lift is ideal in cases requiring elevation of the brow where visible scars are not welcome. It is particularly useful for the aesthetically low brow and those who would benefit from shape change along with elevation, such as the low and flat brow in a female. If dermatochalasis is not severe, it also offers an alternative to upper blepharoplasty and the functionally low brow.

1.3.3 Contraindications

There are no absolute contraindications, only relative ones in terms of performing the procedure. As the instruments are rigid, particularly long foreheads (>9 cm) and convex frontal bones are technically challenging. Though some believe that endoscopic brow lift may lead to hairline elevation, this has not been observed by the senior author. One reason is the controlled posterior dissection.

1.3.4 Results

As with all aesthetic surgery procedures, expectations are key. In the author's personal series of 810 patients [18], revision was required revision in only 20 cases (2.5 %).

1.3.5 Complications

Complications were rare in the author's series [18]. Table 1.2 compares those results with a large-scale survey of American surgeons [19] and a recent review article [20]. It should be noted that the survey of surgeons aggregated data from varying planes.

Table 1.2 Summary of brow lift complications

Complication	Stanek [18], %	Elkwood et al. [19], %	Byun et al. [20], % (95 % CI)
Sensory dysfunction	0	0.6	6.2 (1.1–15.0)
Asymmetry	0.9	1.2	3.6 (1.3–6.8)
Recurrence/revision	1.6	1.8	2.4 (1.1–4.3)
Poor scarring	0	<0.1	1.5 (0.7–2.6)
Motor dysfunction	0	<0.1	1.5 (0.9–2.2)
Hematoma	0.2	<0.1	1 (0.3–1.7)
Infection	2	<0.1	0.4 (0.2–0.8)
Alopecia	3.4	2.9	–
Skin necrosis	0	–	–
Lagophthalmos	0	<0.1	–
Contour	0	<0.1	–

Summary of complications seen in a personal series of 810 [18], an American Society of Plastic Surgeons member survey 19], and weighted complications by percentage derived from systematic review [20]

References

1. Lam VB, Czyx CN, Wulc AE. The brow-eyelid continuum: an anatomic perspective. Clin Plast Surg. 2013;40:1–19.
2. Withey S, Witherow H, Waterhouse N. One hundred cases of endoscopic brow lift. Br J Plast Surg. 2002;55:20–4.
3. Hetzler L, Sykes J. The brow and forehead in periocular rejuvenation. Facial Plast Surg Clin North Am. 2010;18:375–84.
4. Passot R. La chirurgie esthetique des rides du visage. Presse Med. 1919;27:258–62.
5. Hunt HL. Plastic surgery of the head, face and neck. Philadelphia: Lea & Febiger; 1926.
6. Passot R. Chirurgie esthetique pure: techniques et results. Paris: Gaston Doin et Cie; 1930.
7. Fomon S. Surgery of injury and plastic repair. Baltimore: Williams & Wilkins; 1939.
8. Bames HO. Frown disfigurement and ptosis of eyebrows. Plast Reconstr Surg. 1957;19:337–40.
9. Kaye BL. The forehead lift. Plast Reconstr Surg. 1977;60:161–71.
10. Marino H, Gandolfo E. Treatment of forehead wrinkles. Prensa Med Argent. 1964;51:1368–71.
11. Edwards BF. Bilateral temporal neurotomy for frontalis hypermotility. Plast Reconstr Surg. 1957;19:341–5.
12. Viñas JC, Caviglia C, Cortinas JL. Forehead rhytidoplasty and brow lifting. Plast Reconstr Surg. 1976;57:445–54.
13. Pitanguy I. Section of the frontalis-procerus-corrugator aponeurosis in the correction of frontal and glabellar wrinkles. Ann Plast Surg. 1979;2:422–7.
14. Owsley Jr JQ. Cosmetic surgical procedures for the aging face. West J Med. 1982;136:203–10.
15. Vasconez LO. The use of an endoscope in brow lifting. Video presentation at Annual Meeting American Society of Plastic and Reconstructive Surgeons. Washington, DC, 1992.
16. Isse NG. Endoscopic facial rejuvenation: endoforehead, the functional lift. Case reports. Aesthetic Plast Surg. 1994;18:21–9.
17. Ramirez OM, Pozner JN. Laser resurfacing as an adjunct to endoforehead lift, endofacelift and biplanar facelift. Ann Plast Surg. 1997;38:315–21.
18. Stanek JJ, Berry MG. Endoscopic-assisted brow lift: revisions and complications in 810 consecutive cases. J Plast Reconstr Aesthet Surg. 2014;67:998–1016.
19. Elkwood A, Matarasso A, Rankin M, Elkowitz M, Godek CP. National plastic surgery survey: brow lifting techniques and complications. Plast Reconstr Surg. 2001;108:2143–50.
20. Byun S, Mukovozov I, Farrokhyar F, Thoma A. Complications of browlift techniques: a systematic review. Aesthet Surg J. 2013;33:189–200.

2 Minimally Invasive Endoscopic Surgical Treatment of Headache

Edoardo Raposio and Giorgia Caruana

Migraine and tension-type headache are two very common disabling primary disorders [1]. Their high prevalence and great socioeconomic and personal impacts have been widely documented [2]. Although the prevalence and disabling nature of these disorders has roused the interest of many, these conditions remain widely underdiagnosed and undertreated. Many headache sufferers are not helped by standard therapies [3], and the preventive and abortive pharmaceutical agents in use have been related to several adverse effects that are often very onerous.

Literature from the first decade of this century showed a correlation between resection of forehead muscles, occipital muscles, or both and the relief of migraine headaches, renewing notions of the disease's pathogenesis and therapy [4–9]. The theory behind this evidence substantiates the possible role of neuronal hyperexcitability and inflammation involving peripheral craniofacial nerves compressed by surrounding structures such as muscles, blood vessels, or inflamed areas. Authors believe that these nerves may serve as a migraine trigger, and that these trigger points may be eliminated by surgery, thus providing a theoretical therapeutic approach to migraine [7–10]. This theory is better established for migraine than for other types of headache, but it has been shown that surgical treatment of trigger sites may also be beneficial for some non-migraine headaches such as tension-type headaches [11].

Initially, patients who suffered from frontal migraine headache due to muscle compression underwent a procedure developed by Guyuron et al. [12], in which hyperexcitability and inflammation of supraorbital and supratrochlear nerves were eliminated through selective myotomies of depressor supercilii, corrugator supercilii, and procerus muscles, using a transpalpebral approach [13]. Other authors have confirmed that this technique is quite efficient and safe [14, 15], again supporting the trigger-point theory with their surgical outcomes.

At the end of 2005, Walden et al. [16] concluded that a transpalpebral approach did not allow myotomies to be complete, failing to remove more than one third of the corrugator supercilii muscle transverse portion. The whole corrugator supercilii muscle might be removed by means of an endoscopic approach, which was thus claimed to be more thorough and appropriate for this purpose [16]. The use of endoscopic techniques similar to those aimed at rejuvenating the upper third of the aging face [17, 18] also succeeded in improving migraine and tension-type headaches, thus expanding the indications for this surgical approach and the number of procedures potentially covered by plastic surgeons.

This surgical approach [17, 18] is usually performed under general anesthesia. It relies on 3–6 access incisions 1.5–2 cm in length, located 1–2 cm behind the anterior hairline. Two distinct surgical instruments, an endoscope and a dissector, are generally used.

In an effort to reduce the invasiveness of the current endoscopic techniques, we described in 2014 [19, 20] a minimally invasive, endoscopic selective myotomy technique with a single access, performed with a specifically modified endoscope (Karl Storz, Tuttlingen, Germany) and without the need for general anesthesia. In this minimally invasive technique for forehead headache treatment [20], local anesthesia is injected in the forehead, starting from the location of affected nerves (superciliary region) in order to perform an anesthetic block and decrease the pain related to further injections. A single 1.5-cm incision is then performed on the mid-line, behind the frontal hairline, through which skin and frontal muscle are undermined to reach the glabellar region, with the purpose of reaching the insertions of the corrugator supercilii, depressor supercilii, and procerus muscles. Eventually, the endoscope is inserted through the incision and the glabellar muscle group is bilaterally sectioned. At the end of the procedure, the cutaneous access is closed with absorbable suture, without any drainage, and a compressive bandage is positioned all around the patient's head.

E. Raposio, MD, PhD, FICS (✉)
Plastic Surgery Section, Department of Surgical Sciences,
University of Parma, Italy, Via Gramsci 14, Parma 43126, Italy
e-mail: edoardo.raposio@unipr.it

G. Caruana, MD
Department of Surgical Science, Plastic Surgery Section,
Parma University Hospital, Via Gramsci 14, Parma 43126, Italy
e-mail: giorgia.caruana@gmail.com

E. Raposio (ed.), *Atlas of Endoscopic Plastic Surgery*, DOI 10.1007/978-3-319-19461-5_2

2.1 Surgical Technique

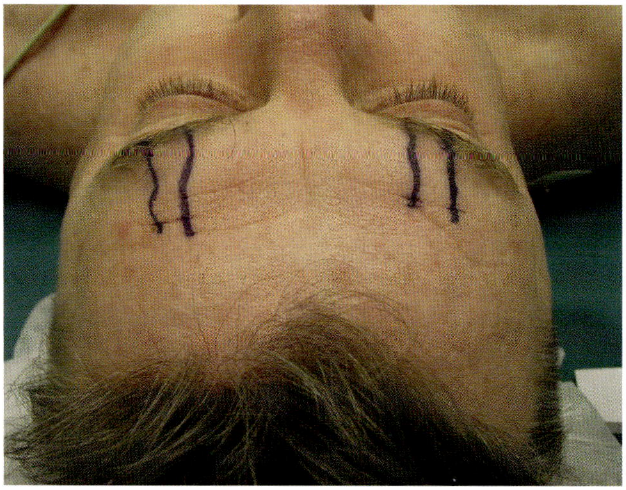

Fig. 2.1 With the patient supine and the head in a neutral position, frontal trigger nerves are located. Skin markings are drawn above the eyebrow bilaterally, at the mid-pupillary line (supraorbital nerve) and 1 cm medially (supratrochlear nerve)

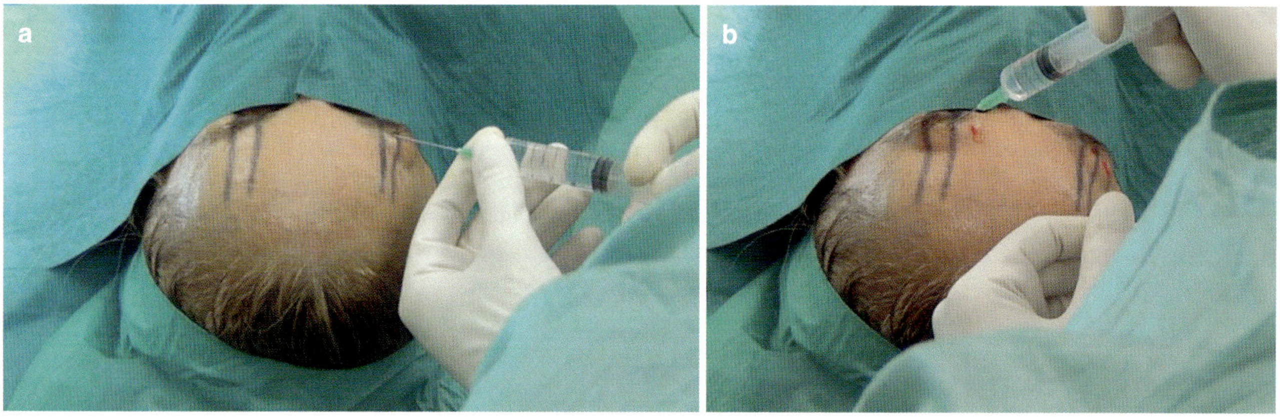

Fig. 2.2 The patient is put under sedo-analgesia and selective supratrochlear and supraorbital nerve block is performed on both on the right side (**a**) and the left side (**b**) in the glabellar region, following the skin markings. This block allows the injection of local anesthetic into the forehead to be completed in a painless manner

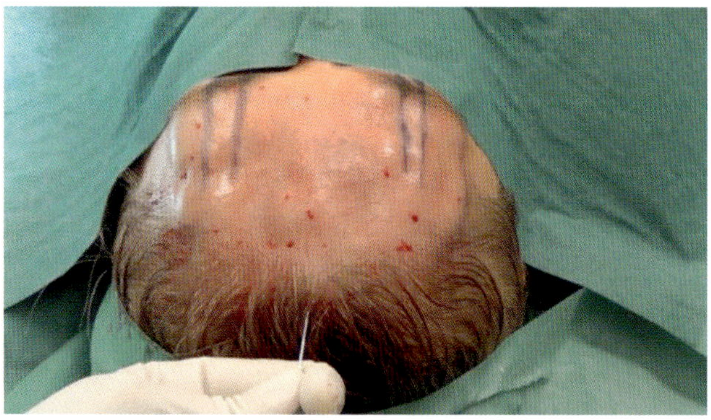

Fig. 2.3 Diluted carbocaine 1 % + 8.4 % sodium bicarbonate are infiltrated throughout the entire forehead, between the glabellar region and about 2 cm behind the anterior hairline. The local anesthetic has a twofold objective: not only anesthesia but also undermining of the tissues and creating a space between the periosteum and adjacent tissues to facilitate endoscopic visualization

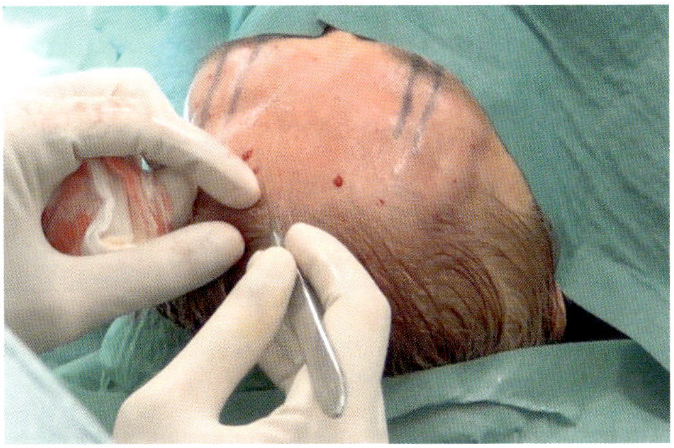

Fig. 2.4 A cutaneous incision 1.5 cm long is performed 1 cm behind the anterior hairline along the midline, dissecting all tissues (cutaneous, subcutaneous, aponeurotic galea) until periosteum is reached in the subgaleal plane. This location is chosen so that the postoperative scar will be hidden in the patient's hair

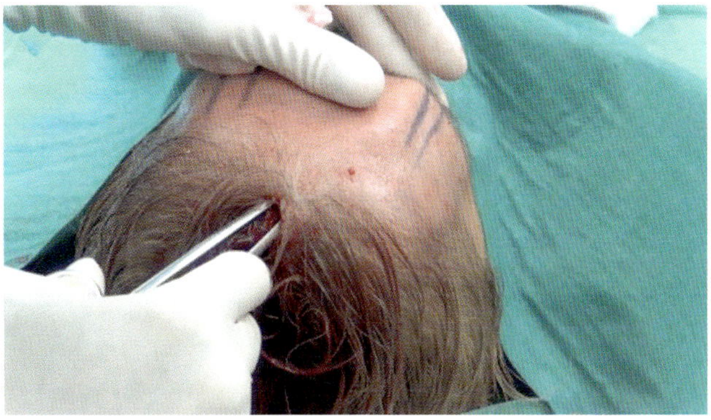

Fig. 2.5 Facilitated by the previous injection of local anesthetic, tissues all over the forehead bilaterally are undermined in the subgaleal plane through the hairline incision by means of long scissors. Undermining must be done carefully, particularly when the inferior limit of the undermining area (superciliary region) is reached, in order not to damage supratrochlear and supraorbital nerves. The lateral anatomic limit of the undermining area is the temporal region, bilaterally

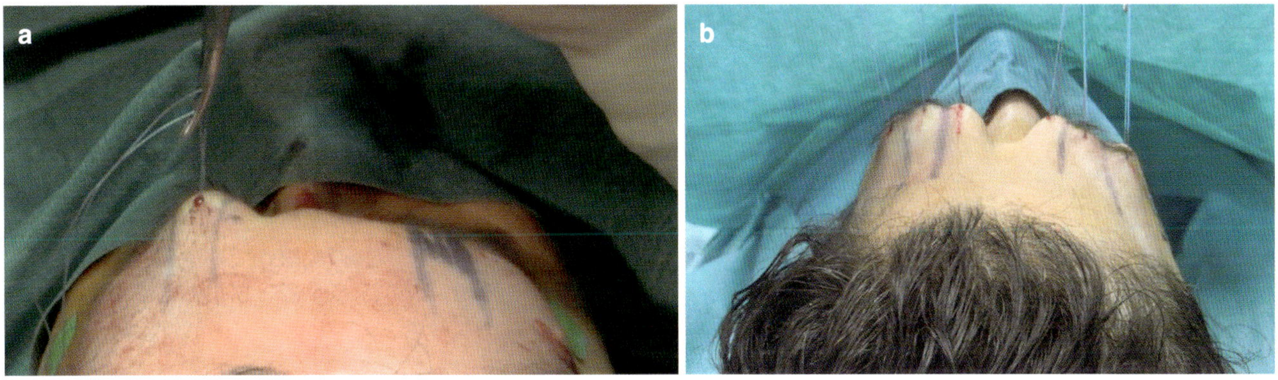

Fig. 2.6 (**a**, **b**), Nylon 1–0 sutures are placed in the superciliary region at each side of both supratrochlear and supraorbital nerves bilaterally, with the purpose of lifting the frontal skin during the endoscopic procedure and better visualizing the anatomic structures

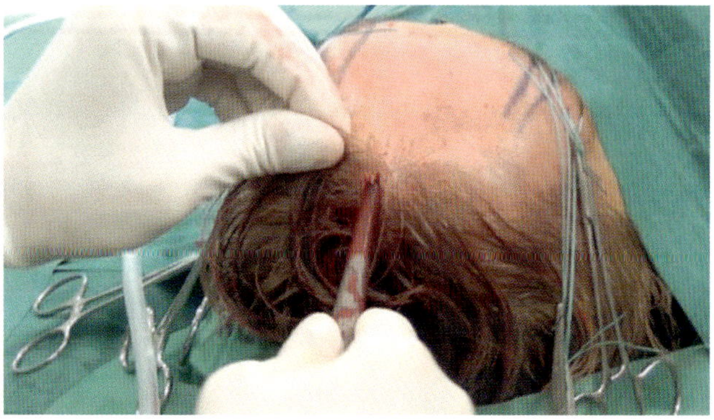

Fig. 2.7 To clean the subgaleal plane of blood and residual anesthetic fluid, suction of the entire undermined forehead is performed through the hairline incision before inserting the endoscope and whenever the endoscopic view is not clear

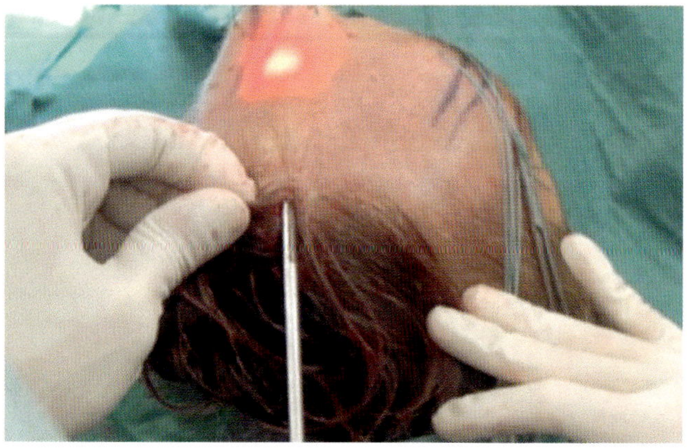

Fig. 2.8 The endoscope is inserted through the incision in the subgaleal plane until the superciliary region is reached, in order to perform the section of the corrugator supercilii, depressor supercilii, and procerus muscles bilaterally, thus decompressing the supraorbital and supratrochlear nerves bilaterally. Our modified endoscope (Karl Storz, Tuttlingen, Germany) consists of a 9-mm trocar with an air/insufflator/suction triple valve, a straight Hopkins telescope with fiber-light transmission, a Wittmöser operating sheath with a connection for high-frequency diathermy, and a specifically designed, elliptical-tipped wire loop electrode for electrocautery

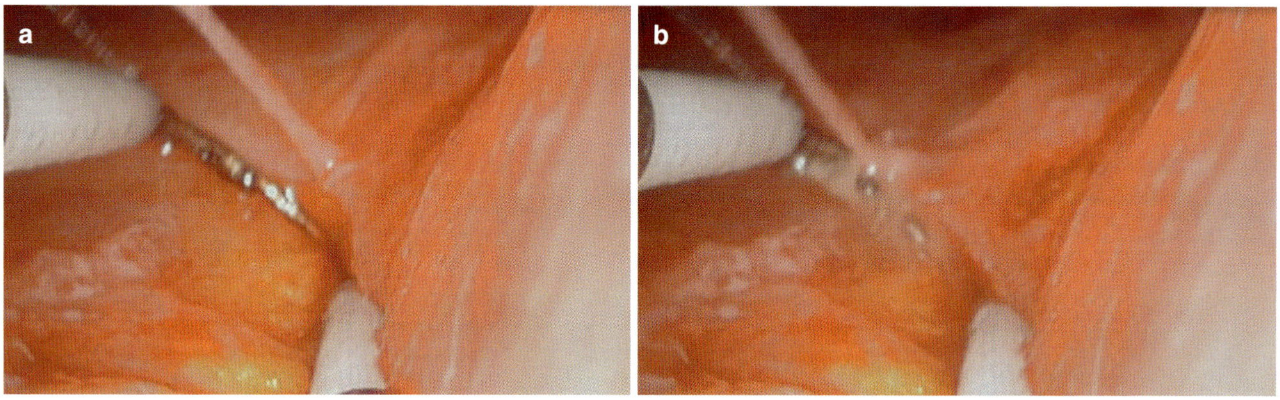

Fig. 2.9 The modified endoscope is used to perform endoscopically assisted section of the corrugator supercilii, depressor supercilii, and procerus muscles bilaterally, with the purpose of decompressing the supraorbital nerve, which is not injured during dissection. During this procedure, it is important to dissect every part of the muscle, which receives facial nerve fibers responsible for contraction of the muscle itself, in order to prevent irritation to surrounding nerves from the muscle's movement. In these figures, the left supraorbital nerve is recognizable before (**a**) and during (**b**) the dissection; it is located in the superciliary region, 1 cm medial to the mid-pupillary line

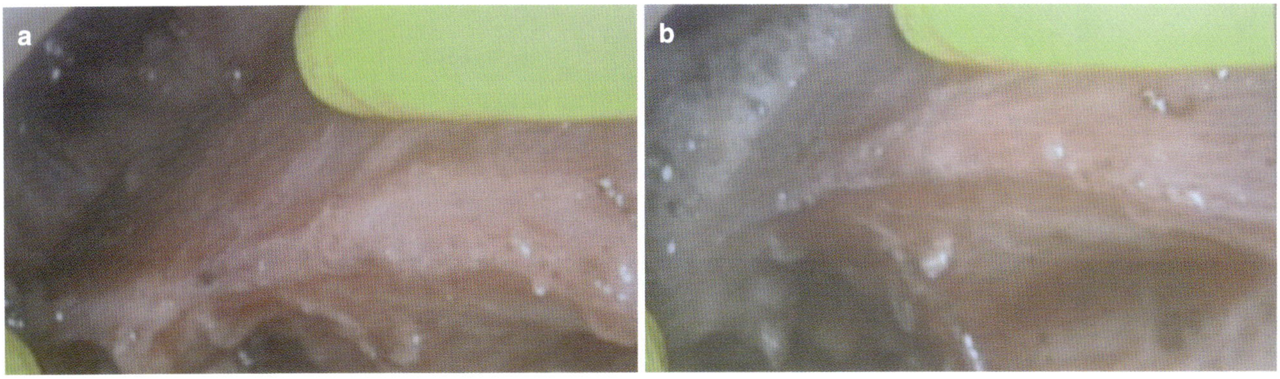

Fig. 2.10 Right supratrochlear nerve before (**a**) and during (**b**) the endoscopically assisted section of the right corrugator supercilii muscle. The supratrochlear nerve is located in the superciliary region, about 1.75 cm from the midline. Sections of glabellar muscles are performed at each side of both the supratrochlear and supraorbital nerves bilaterally. Endoscopic visualization is helpful in avoiding injury to the nerves and better identifying the muscles

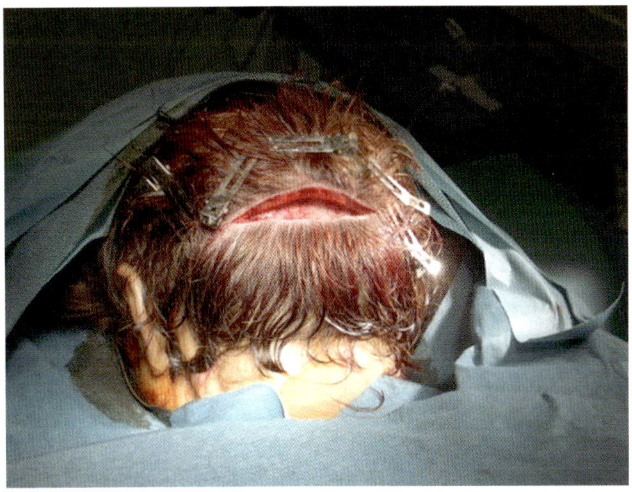

Fig. 2.11 Surgical treatment of migraine and tension-type headache is also a useful procedure for occipital headaches, but headaches of this type require open surgery. In this patient, trigger sites have been identified in the greater occipital nerve (GON) bilaterally. Therefore, after performing local anesthesia, a horizontal occipital scalp incision 6 cm in length is performed along the superior nuchal midline to expose subcutaneous structures. No trichotomy is needed, and the scar from the incision will be hidden in the patient's hair

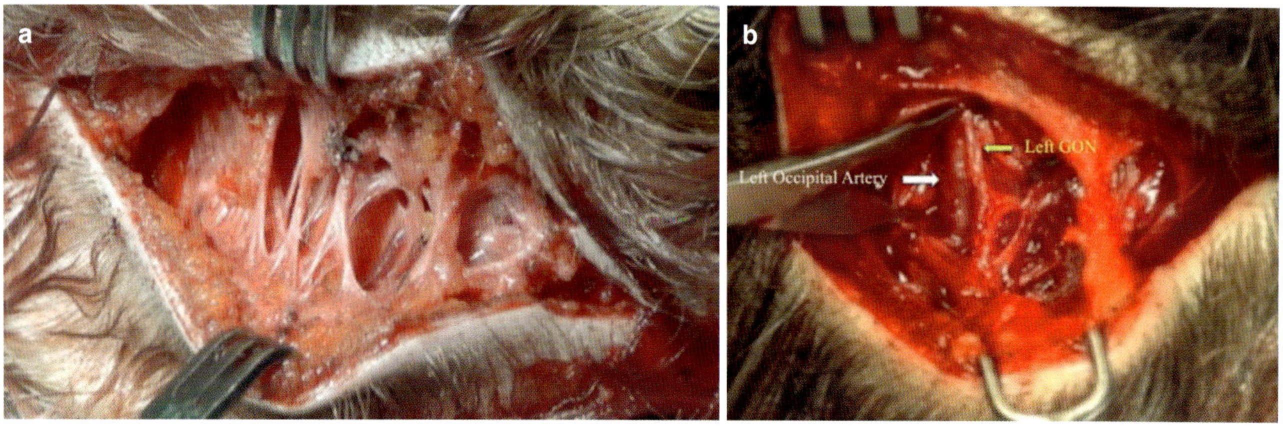

Fig. 2.12 For occipital headaches with the GON as the main trigger bilaterally, the occipital muscle is dissected first, then trapezius fibers are divided and the muscle is minutely undermined, thus exposing the GON and the semispinalis capitis muscle, which is also undermined, following the nerve course as far as possible (**a**). The GON is then isolated from the splenius capitis muscle, which is located laterally behind it, and from the occipital vascular bundle. Sometimes the occipital artery may be more distended than expected; its pulsing activity might be the cause of nerve irritation (**b**)

Conclusions

Before considering this type of surgery, it is essential that each patient meets the criteria for migraine and tension-type headache as set forth by the International Classification of Headache Disorders II (ICHD-II) [21]. Surgical treatment of headache is indicated for patients who are in good health and have experienced 15 or more frontal migraine headaches without aura (ICHD-II: 1.1), tension-type headaches (ICHD-II: 2.3), or new daily persistent headaches each month (ICHD-II: 4.8) [20]. Patients who do not benefit from any medications for their headache are also eligible for the surgery. Patients with cluster headache (ICHD-II: 3), episodic tension-type headache (ICHD-II: 2.1, 2.2), or secondary headaches are considered ineligible for this type of treatment [21].

At the first meeting with the surgeon, a detailed evaluation is performed to confirm the frequency, duration, and intensity of the headaches and to identify the most common focal (trigger) site of onset. Patients are then asked to complete a comprehensive headache questionnaire before the surgery and at least 6 months after the surgery, in order to evaluate the effectiveness of the surgical procedure, the degree of reduction in pain and medication use, the eventual onset of new symptoms, or any adverse effect. Written informed consent must be obtained from all patients before surgery.

After surgery, patients usually report some degree of frontal numbness, which lasts for about 2–3 months and then disappears definitively. Some patients (20 %), depending on differences in cutaneous thickness, may present 1-cm frontal cutaneous scars, as a result of thermal injury in the region of the glabellar muscles. Hair thinning at the site of the endoscopic incision also may be observed, though it is infrequent (13.3 %). This thinning might be partially avoided by performing the scalp incision parallel to the orientation of the hair follicles.

A 5-year follow-up of surgical treatment of migraine headache has been described in literature [22], showing that 88 % of patients received benefit from the surgery (29 % reporting complete elimination of migraine headache and 59 % reporting a significant decrease in their attacks). No significant change was reported by 12 %.

After 2 years of follow-up, the minimally invasive approach yielded a total positive response of 93 %: 33 % of patients reported complete elimination of their attacks and 60 % experienced significant improvement (at least 50 % reduction in intensity or frequency). Only 7 % did not notice a change in their headaches. Considering these data and the lack of major complications from the operation, endoscopic surgical treatment of migraine or tension-type headache can be considered a valid alternative to pharmacological treatment, especially for those patients who do not benefit from those therapies or who have experienced serious adverse effects [20].

References

1. Olesen J, Steiner TJ. The International classification of headache disorders, 2nd edn (ICDH-II). J Neurol Neurosurg Psychiatry. 2004;75:808–11.
2. Lipton RB, Bigal ME, Diamond M, Freitag F, Reed ML, Stewart WF. AMPP Advisory Group. Migraine prevalence, disease burden, and the need for preventive therapy. Neurology. 2007;68:343–9.
3. Dodick DW. Triptan nonresponder studies: implications for clinical practice. Headache. 2005;45:156–62.
4. Guyuron B, Varghai A, Michelow BJ, Thomas T, Davis J. Corrugator supercilii muscle resection and migraine headaches. Plast Reconstr Surg. 2000;106:429–34.
5. Mosser SW, Guyuron B, Janis JE, Rohrich RJ. The anatomy of the greater occipital nerve: Implications for the etiology of migraine headaches. Plast Reconstr Surg. 2004;113:693–7.
6. Dash KS, Janis JE, Guyuron B. The lesser and third occipital nerves and migraine headaches. Plast Reconstr Surg. 2005;115:1752–8.
7. Janis JE, Dhanik A, Howard JH. Validation of trigger point theory of migraine headaches: Single-surgeon experience using Botulinum toxin and surgical decompression. Plast Reconstr Surg. 2011;128:123–31.
8. Guyuron B, Tucker T, Davis J. Surgical treatment of migraine headaches. Headache. 2003;43:302–3.
9. Guyuron B, Reed D, Friegler JS, Davis J, Pashmini N, Amini S. A placebo controlled surgical trial for the treatment of migraine headaches. Plast Reconstr Surg. 2009;124:461–8.
10. Malick A, Burstein R. Peripheral and central sensitization during migraine. Funct Neurol. 2000;15 Suppl 3:28–35.
11. Bearden WH, Anderson RL. Corrugator superciliaris muscle excision for tension and migraine headaches. Ophthal Plast Reconstr Surg. 2005;21:418–22.
12. Guyuron B, Kriegler JS, Davis J, Amini SB. Comprehensive surgical treatment of migraine headaches. Plast Reconstr Surg. 2005;115:1–9.
13. Guyuron B, Knize DM. Corrugator supercilii resection through blepharoplasty incision. Plast Reconstr Surg. 2001;107:606–7.
14. Dirnberger F, Becker K. Surgical treatment of migraine headaches by corrugator muscle resection. Plast Reconstr Surg. 2004;114:652–7.
15. Poggi JT, Grizzel BE, Helmer SD. Confirmation of surgical decompression to relieve migraine headaches. Plast Reconstr Surg. 2008;122:115–22.
16. Walden JL, Brown CC, Klapper AJ, Chia CT, Aston SJ. An anatomical comparison of transpalpebral, endoscopic and coronal approaches to demonstrate exposure and extent of brow depressor muscle resection. Plast Reconstr Surg. 2005;116:1479–87.
17. Abramo AC, Dorta AA. Selective myotomy in forehead endoscopy. Plast Reconstr Surg. 2003;112:873–9.
18. Papadopulos NA, Eder M, Weigand C, Biemer E, Kovacs L. A review of 13 years of experience with endoscopic forehead-lift. Arch Facial Plast Surg. 2012;14:336–41.
19. Caruana G, Bertozzi N, Boschi E, Grieco MP, Grignaffini E, Raposio E. Endoscopic forehead surgery for migraine therapy: personal technique. Ann Ital Chir. 2014;85:583–6.
20. Raposio E, Caruana G. Frontal endoscopic myotomies for chronic headache. J Craniofac Surg. 2015;26(3):e201–3.
21. Headache Classification Committee of the International Headache Society. Classification and diagnostic criteria for headache disorders, cranial neuralgias and facial pain. Cephalalgia. 1988;8 Suppl 7:1–96.
22. Guyuron B, Kriegler J, Davis J, Amini SB. Five-year outcome of surgical treatment of migraine headaches. Plast Reconstr Surg. 2011;127:603–8.

Endoscopic Harvest of the Fascia Lata for Facial Reanimation

3

Paul M. Rea and Stephen Morley

Fascia lata is a band of tissue that comprises the deep fascia of the lower limb. It is attached superiorly to the sacrum and coccyx and laterally to the iliac crest. Anteriorly, the fascia lata is attached to the inguinal ligament and the superior ramus of the pubis. Medially it is attached to the ischium, the sacrotuberous ligament, and the inferior ramus of the pubis. The fascia lata becomes thickened over the lateral aspect of the thigh, forming the iliotibial tract. At its upper portion, it splits into the small tensor fasciae latae. Inferiorly, the iliotibial tract is attached to the lateral condyle of the tibia. Inferior to this, the fascia lata is attached to all bony aspects of the knee joint.

As such, the fascia lata is superficial, making it easy to access surgically. It is a tough, highly collagenated sheath [1] with fibers that run parallel to the axis of the lower limb [2]. It is relatively avascular and has a large surface area and an incredibly high tensile strength, making it ideal for use in static reconstructive surgery [3]. It has been used for many years in a variety of surgical procedures, especially static facial reanimation [2, 4–6]. The use of autogenous tissue avoids issues arising from the use of synthetic materials or donor tissue, including infection, granuloma formation, extrusion, or even late-stage failure of the material transferred [7–9].

Conventionally, fascia lata has been accessed by a single, large incision on the lateral thigh, or by two or even three longitudinal incisions [10]. With a single large incision, unsightly scarring will be present, with a detrimental cosmetic effect [2, 6, 11, 12]. The use of two or three incisions is effectively a blind dissection of the graft tissue, not allowing for clear visualisation of the fascia lata for harvesting [6, 13].

A variety of other techniques have been developed for accessing fascia lata, including the use of strippers and fasciotomies, as well as smaller incisions [6, 14]. Endoscopic techniques have been receiving attention for retrieving the fascia lata. As endoscopes are typically used in cosmetic procedures such as breast augmentation, facial rejuvenation, and orthopaedic operations [15, 16], their use seems a viable option.

Tucker et al. [17] successfully used an endoscopic technique to harvest fascia lata for the repair of a recurrent ventral hernia. They inserted a 10-mm endoscope via a small incision on the lower lateral thigh. Using insufflation and electrocautery, a sheet of fascia lata measuring 12 × 15 cm was successfully retrieved. Another approach to endoscopic harvesting was used by Malhotra et al. [18], who used a 4-mm rigid 30° endoscope to retrieve fascia lata measuring 10–12 cm via two incisions on the lateral aspect of the thigh. The proximal and distal incisions permitted sufficient access to harvest the fascia lata for brow lift and lower eye sling surgical interventions.

More recently, Rea et al. [19] have shown that endoscopic access to the fascia lata is perfectly feasible not only in the cadaver but also in the operative environment. They showed that the fascia lata could be harvested not only via two small incisions (one distal and the other proximal) on the lateral aspect of the thigh, but also via a single, proximal incision. This technique clearly minimises cosmetic effects on the patient's thigh while achieving adequate tissue retrieval.

P.M. Rea, MBChB, MSc, DipFMS, FHEA, PhD, MIMI, RMIP, FRSA (✉)
Laboratory of Human Anatomy, Room 349, School of Life Sciences, College of Medical, Veterinary, and Life Sciences, University of Glasgow, Glasgow G12 8QQ, UK
e-mail: Paul.Rea@glasgow.ac.uk

S. Morley, MD, FRCS (Plast)
Canniesburn Plastic Surgery Unit, Glasgow Royal Infirmary, Jubilee Building, 84 Castle Street, Glasgow G4 0SF, UK
e-mail: Stephen.Morley@ggc.scot.nhs.uk

E. Raposio (ed.), *Atlas of Endoscopic Plastic Surgery*, DOI 10.1007/978-3-319-19461-5_3

3.1 Indications for the Use of Fascia Lata

Fascia lata can be used for a variety of surgical interventions. It has been used for reconstruction of the anterior skull-base dura when it is accessed for resection of tumours or repair of defects (e.g., in fronto-naso-orbital or skull-base fractures) and when repair of a cerebrospinal fistula is required [20, 21]. Indeed, the use of fascia lata has been popular in many craniofacial procedures. It is typically used in the correction of lid, orbital, and facial deformities, including rhytidectomy, cheiloplasty, blepharoplasty, brow lift, and soft tissue procedures [5, 10, 22, 23]. The use of fascia lata in static facial reanimation is becoming increasingly popular [4, 24].

In addition, the fascia lata has proved beneficial in reconstruction of the knee, including the anterior cruciate ligament [25, 26], as well as for sacrocolpopexy procedures in women with vaginal vault prolapse after hysterectomy [27, 28]. It has also shown great durability and viability in a variety of urological procedures to maintain continence [29, 30] and in the reconstruction of abdominal wall and groin defects, along with its related muscle [17, 31].

Fascia lata is ideal for autogenous transfer because of its great tensile strength, maintenance of presurgical length, and the fact that it incorporates well into surrounding tissue [4, 13]. The resistance of the fascia lata has been cited as approximately 3266 N, making it at least as strong as some of the synthetic materials currently available [25]. The traditional open access approach to the fascia lata created a number of problems, however, including unsightly scarring on the lateral aspect of the thigh, postoperative haemorrhage, pain when walking, wound pain, and limping [12, 32]. If a large portion of fascia lata was harvested, muscle herniation could also occur [33].

With the growing popularity of the endoscope in various surgical procedures, including ophthalmic and plastic reconstruction [17, 18], it seems sensible as an ideal mechanism for harvesting fascia lata. Early studies of endoscopic access to the fascia lata reported good illumination; enhanced magnification at the site; and no hematoma, muscle herniation, or any other morbidity [17, 18] (Figs. 3.1, 3.2, 3.3, and 3.4). Despite initial concern that operative time would be longer with endoscopic retrieval of the fascia lata than with the traditional open technique, the difference was shown not to be significant [19].

Fascia lata is now commonly used to provide static facial support in cases of facial paralysis. When the facial nerve has little or no function, the mid face develops ptosis or sagging and the modiolus tends to droop. The result is an asymmetrical facial position at rest and oral incompetence, which cause great distress for the patient in regards to facial appearance and function. The affected side of the face can be lifted and supported by placing fascia lata slings under the skin to suspend the modiolus to a suitable support, usually the zygoma. Other indications for fascia lata grafts include revision of other surgical procedures used to reanimate the paralysed face, such as if a free muscle transfer has been used to "dynamise" a paralysed face but the position of the modiolus has slipped or was not sufficiently lifted. In these cases, a strip of fascia lata can be placed over the muscle to provide additional lift at the modiolus. Using an endoscopic approach for fascia lata harvest, strips of fascia up to 14×3 cm—a size easily sufficient for the technique of static facial slings—can be harvested from two small access incisions [19].

With no complications, reduced morbidity, and no scarring, it appears that the endoscopic approach to the fascia lata seems sensible to adopt into routine surgical procedures when access to this tissue is needed. For patients who are immunocompromised, elderly, or unable to undergo numerous operations, the use of autogenous fascia lata is ideal [4, 26]. With minimal scarring and no morbidity associated with endoscopic access, the ideal operative situation has been achieved [17–19].

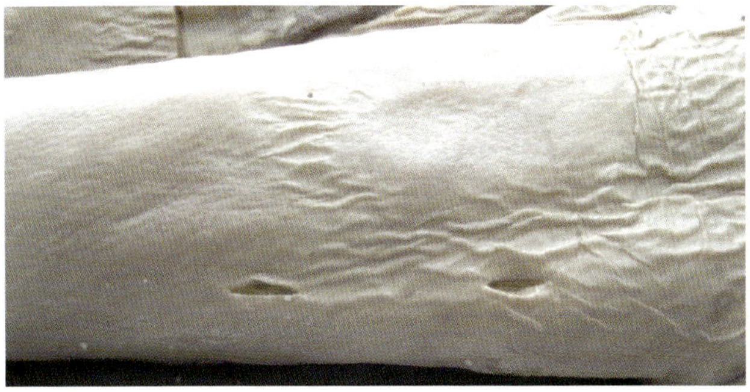

Fig. 3.1 Proximal and distal skin incisions on the cadaver's left thigh during experimental work undertaken to demonstrate the feasibility of endoscopic access for harvesting of fascia lata (*Image courtesy of* Mr. Stuart McNally.)

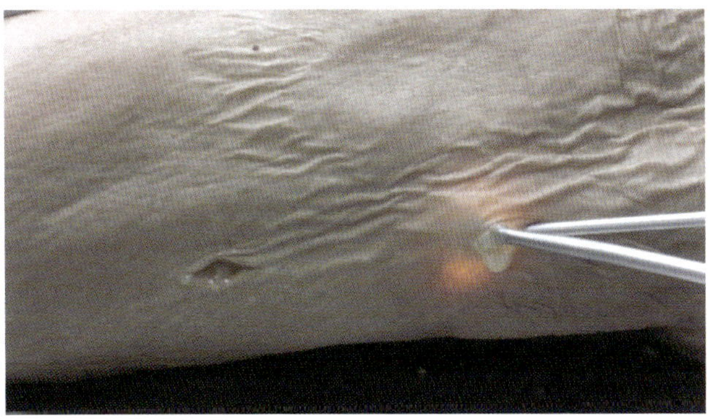

Fig. 3.2 Retrieval of the fascia lata using an optical dissector (*Image courtesy of* Mr. Stuart McNally.)

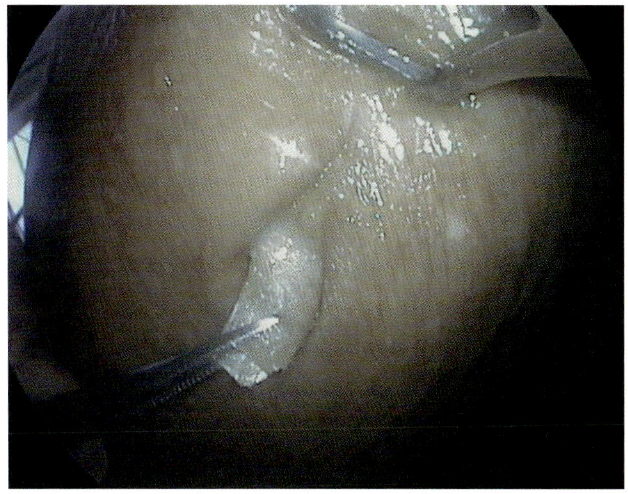

Fig. 3.3 Retrieval of the fascia lata strip through the proximal skin incision (*Image courtesy of* Mr. Stuart McNally.)

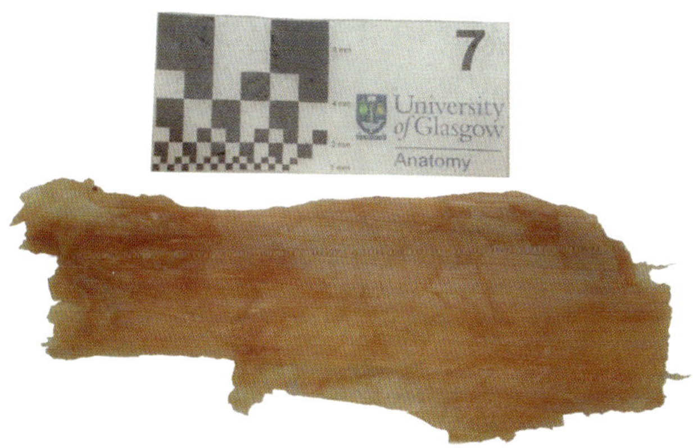

Fig. 3.4 Fascia lata taken from the cadaver in determining feasibility of endoscopic access for retrieval of the tissue. The scale bars include 1, 2, 4, and 8 mm and 1 cm. The maximum amount of fascia lata tissue retrieved during the experimental procedure was initially 90×30 mm (*Image courtesy of* Mr. Stuart McNally.)

3.2 Contraindications for the Use of Fascia Lata

The fascia lata should not be accessed for use in any reconstructive procedure if there has been previous trauma to the fascia lata or surgical retrieval of it. It is always pertinent to consider surgically accessing a site far away from the site that needs to be operated on. It may be easier to use temporalis fascia, especially on facial procedures like ptosis surgery. Surgery should not be performed until any infection at the site is satisfactorily treated [34].

3.3 Complications

Table 3.1 summarises the complications that can arise when traditional open access to the fascia lata is attempted, and lists relevant discussions of these pathologies. Endoscopic access to fascia lata, on the other hand, produces no major complications. The very slight prolongation of operating time is likely to disappear when surgical teams have more experience with endoscopic access to the fascia lata. With the lack of morbidity after the procedure, it makes sense to undertake the harvesting of the fascia lata by the endoscopic approach.

Table 3.1 Complications of open access to Fascia Lata

Complication	References
Reduction in muscle power	Amir et al. [13]
Visible scarring	Wheatcroft et al. [12] Amir et al. [13] Leibovitch et al. [2] Zandi [11] Kashkouli [6]
Wound pain	Barron and Saad [32] Wheatcroft et al. [12]
Limping/weakness of harvested side	Dubiel and Wigren [33] Wheatcroft et al. [12]
Bleeding	Dubiel and Wigren [33]
Wound dehiscence	Amir et al. [13]
Muscle herniation	Dubiel and Wigren [33]

3.4 Surgical Technique

The surgery is performed under general or regional anaesthesia with the patient in the supine position. For the harvest of fascia lata, a solution of local anaesthetic and adrenaline is infused around the upper, outer thigh in a volume depending on the amount of tissue to be harvested. The endoscope used to perform the procedure in all cases was the Karl Storz HOPKINS® II Wide Angle Forward-Oblique Telescope (30°, 4 mm diameter, 18 cm length), and visual feedback was provided by a Karl-Storz Endoscope Tele Pack™ at 3× magnification.

Two 1- to 2-cm lazy-S skin incisions are made approximately 10 cm apart on the lateral aspect of the donor thigh. If the length of graft required is 5 cm or less, a single incision can be made. Using small retractors, dissection is made deeply to expose the fibres of the fascia lata, which should be clearly visualised as a tough, glistening layer in the base of the surgical field (Figs. 3.3, 3.5 and 3.6).

A subcutaneous pocket is developed over the fascia to be harvested. This plane is usually fairly avascular, but bipolar cautery is used if required. Through the upper skin incision, a 2- to 3-cm incision of the underlying fascia lata is made perpendicular to the skin. Passing under the fascia lata on the proximal side, it is separated from the underlying vastus lateralis by using an optical dissector attachment such as a Karl Storz TAKE-APART® elevator and Karl Storz CLICKLINE® scissors (Fig. 3.7). It is also separated from the overlying subcutaneous tissue by the same means. Using the endoscope for visualisation, the fascia lata is cut, ensuring a strip 2–3 cm wide all the way to the region of the distal skin incision for the desired length. The separated rectangular fascia lata strip, is then removed through the distal skin incision using fine forceps. Haemostasis is achieved using the endoscope and bipolar cautery.

The graft is defatted using scissors, and the recipient bed is prepared. If the graft is to be used as a primary static support, the length required is 12–13 cm. For revisionary procedures, a shorter length is often sufficient.

In the cheek, the local anaesthetic and adrenaline solution is infused subcutaneously. A pre-auricular, post-tragal incision is made and a tunnel is developed in the deep subcutaneous tissues. A small nasolabial incision of (1.5–2 cm) is made and the sub-cutaneous pocket is developed to communicate with this incision. If lip support is also required, the pocket is developed behind the vermillion of the upper and lower lip to the midpoint of the mouth or slightly beyond. Small incisions (5 mm) are made in the upper and lower lip.

The fascia is secured distally with sutures and fixed proximally to the zygomatic arch using a bone anchor (Fig. 3.8). Fixation to the temporoparietal fascia is also possible but is less secure. The aim of the fascial positioning is to achieve a slight overcorrection of the position of the modiolus during the operative procedure, to allow for some postoperative stretch of the graft and relaxation of the face (Figs. 3.9 and 3.10).

The time of endoscopic harvest averages 20 min, no longer than the typical open technique previously used. Complications related to the donor site using this technique are no higher than in an open approach. Potential complications include bleeding, infection at the donor or recipient site, and bulging or herniation of the vastus lateralis muscle through the resulting defects in the fascia lata.

The principle advantage to the patient with the endoscopic technique is shorter scars. The surgeon achieves an optimal view of the operating field. The typical scarring related to fascia lata harvest using a standard open technique would be a double 4-cm scar. Using an endoscopic assist, this scarring is typically either a single scar of 2–3 cm or two scars of 2 cm. This difference is particularly important in younger patients, where minimising scarring is an advantage.

When only a single incision is performed for endoscopic access, it is up to 75 % smaller than the incision used to perform an open procedure. In addition, there are no complications related to the donor site where endoscopic retrieval was undertaken. Endoscopic harvest of the fascia lata has been shown to be practical and straightforward, using a minimum of specialist equipment. The procedure lends itself to an endoscopic approach and is likely to gain widespread acceptance with improvements in instrumentation.

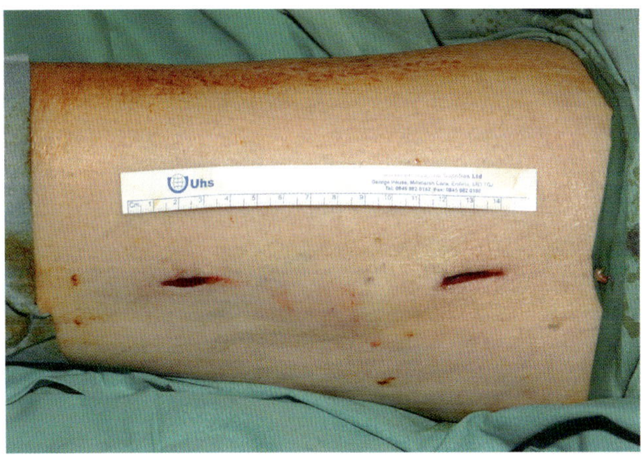

Fig. 3.5 Proximal (*right*) and distal (*left*) skin incisions carried out in the initial approach to access the fascia lata using the endoscopic technique in the operative environment

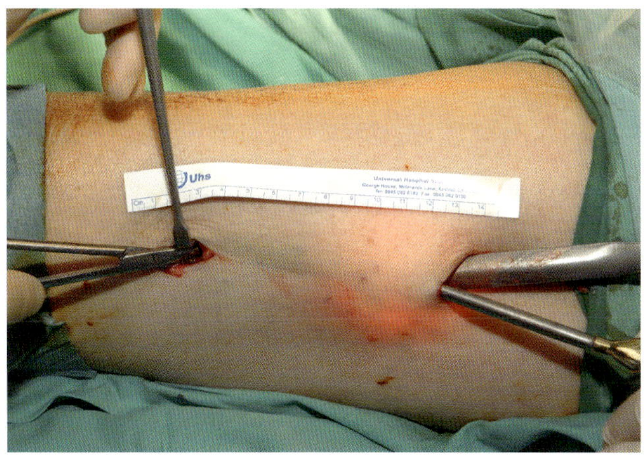

Fig. 3.7 Dissection proceeds using an endoscopic dissector in combination with scissors, with endoscopic assistance

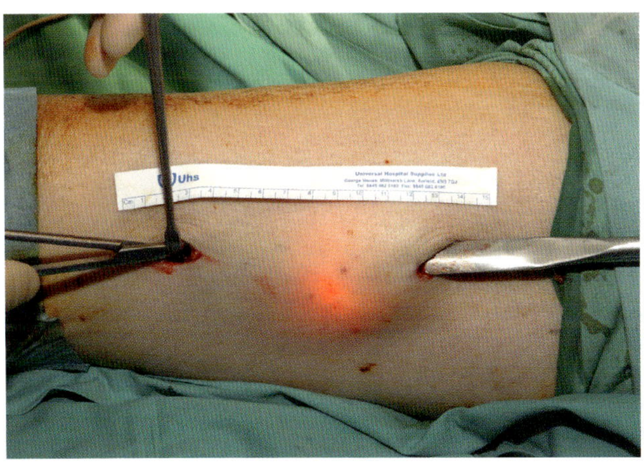

Fig. 3.6 Subcutaneous dissection over superficial aspect of the fascia lata, facilitated by an endoscope inserted into the proximal access incision

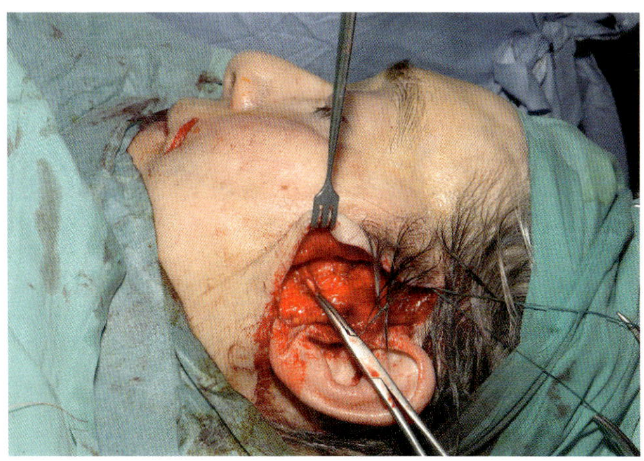

Fig. 3.8 The fascia lata strip has been secured to the upper and lower lip and is fixed to the zygoma under appropriate tension

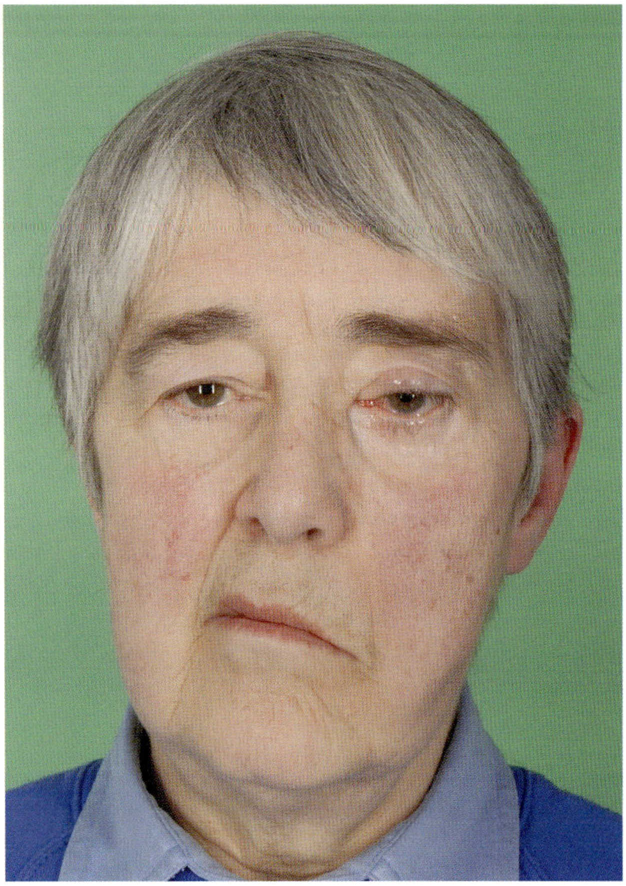

Fig. 3.9 73-year-old female patient with a left-sided facial palsy following melanoma removal (*From* Rea et al. [19], with permission of Springer Science + Business Media; © 2013 Springer-Verlag.)

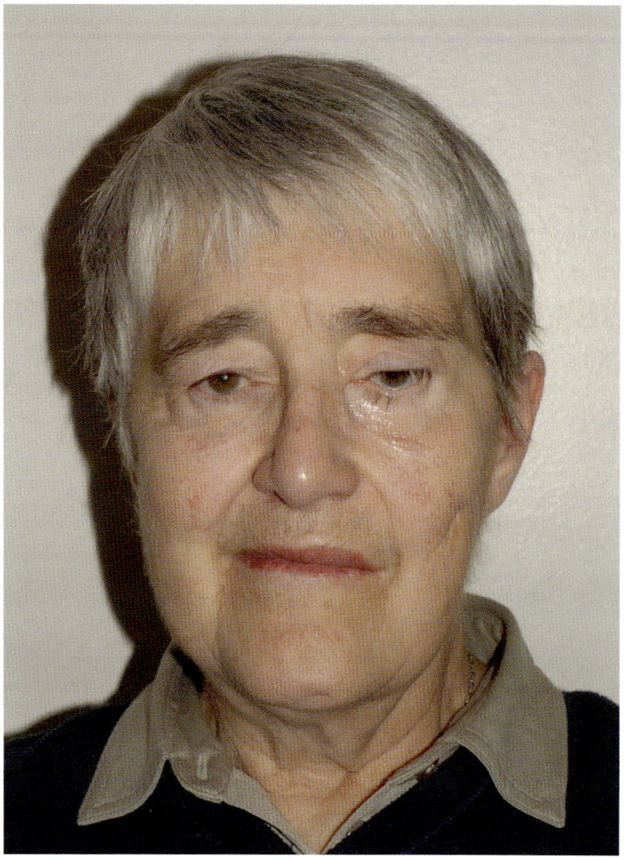

Fig. 3.10 The same patient 6 months after surgery, following successful endoscopic access to fascia lata and facial reanimation (*From* Rea et al. [19], with permission of Springer Science + Business Media; © 2013 Springer-Verlag.)

Conclusions

For reconstructive purposes, autogenous tissue is preferable to donor tissue or synthetic materials, as it will not be rejected and is not prone to problems such as granulomas, extrusion, or infection [7, 9, 34–37].

Endoscopic access to the fascia lata permits harvesting of an adequate size of tissue. Tucker et al. [17] were able to successfully harvest a strip of tissue up to 12×15 cm for ventral hernia repairs. Similarly, Malhotra et al. [18] retrieved a strip of fascia lata measuring 10–12 cm via a single incision at either the proximal or distal aspect of the thigh. Rea et al. [19] performed endoscopic access on several patients and were able to harvest fascia lata strips measuring up to 14×2.5 cm via a single incision (or at most two, one proximal and one distal) on the thigh. Rea et al. [19] also recorded no postoperative complications. Compared with the previous large incisions and their high incidence of postoperative morbidity, endoscopic access for harvesting the fascia lata seems the sensible option to retrieve this tissue, from both a cosmetic and functional perspective.

References

1. Drever JM. A simple method for obtaining fascia lata grafts. Plast Reconstr Surg. 1972;50:196–7.
2. Leibovitch I, Leibovitch L, Dray JP. Long-term results of frontalis suspension using autogenous fascia lata for congenital ptosis in children under 3 years of age. Am J Ophthalmol. 2003;136:866–71.
3. Sclafani AP, McCormick SA, Cocker R. Biophysical and microscopic analysis of homologous dermal and fascial materials for facial aesthetic and reconstructive uses. Arch Facial Plast Surg. 2002;4:164–71.
4. Barret J, McDowell F, Fryer MP. Facial paralysis supported with autogenous fascia lata. Ann Surg. 1947;127:858–62.
5. Rose EH. Autogenous fascia lata grafts: clinical applications in reanimation of the totally or partially paralyzed face. Plast Reconstr Surg. 2005;116:20–32.
6. Kashkouli MB. A novel technique for small-incision fascia lata harvesting without a fasciatome for the frontalis suspension procedure. Orbit. 2007;26:203–6.
7. Leone CR, Shore JW, Van Gemert JV. Silicone rod frontalis sling for the correction of blepharoptosis. Ophthalmic Surg. 1981;12:881–7.
8. Zweep HP, Spauwen PH. Evaluation of expanded polytetrafluoroethylene (e-PTFE) and autogenous fascia lata in frontalis suspension. A comparative clinical study. Acta Chir Plast. 1992;34:129–37.
9. Manners RM, Tyers AG, Morris RJ. The use of Prolene as a temporary suspensory material for brow suspension in young children. Eye. 1994;8:346–8.
10. Bilgin LK, Yeniad B. The long-term results of frontalis suspension using autogenous fascia lata in children with congenital ptosis under 3 years old. Plast Surg Int. 2010;2010:609462. doi:10.1155/2010/609462.
11. Zandi A. Harvesting fascia lata from brow suspension procedure via two small skin incisions. J Res Med Sci. 2006;11:396–9.
12. Wheatcroft SM, Vardy SJ, Tyers AG. Complications of fascia lata harvesting for ptosis surgery. Br J Ophthalmol. 1997;81:581–3.
13. Amir A, Gatot A, Zucker G, Sagi A, Fliss DM. Harvesting large fascia lata sheaths: a rational approach. Skull Base Surg. 2000;10:29–34.
14. Bhatti A, Soueid AM, Baden JM. Fascia lata harvesting: minimal access for maximum harvest. A new technique. Plast Reconstr Surg. 2010;126:277–88e.
15. Ramirez OM. Endoscopic techniques in facial rejuvenation: an overview. Part I. Aesthetic Plast Surg. 1994;18:141–7.
16. Deporter M, Kerpel WD. Reanimation of the paralyzed face by entire temporalis muscle transposition. An endoscopic approach. Eur J Plast Surg. 2004;28:190–4.
17. Tucker JG, Choat D, Zubowicz VN. Videoscopically assisted fascia lata harvest for the correction of recurrent ventral hernia. South Med J. 1997;90:399–401.
18. Malhotra R, Selva D, Olver JM. Endoscopic harvesting of autogenous fascia lata. Ophthal Plast Reconstr Surg. 2007;23:372–5.
19. Rea P, Welsh E, Morley S. Endoscopic access to fascia lata for use in static facial reanimation – a cadaveric and clinical study. Eur J Plast Surg. 2013;36:673–8.
20. Fliss DM, Zucker G, Cohen A, Amir A, Sagi A, Rosenberg L, et al. Early outcome and complications of the extended subcranial approach to the anterior skull base. Laryngoscope. 1999;109:153–60.
21. Amenta PS, Lynn M, Kenning T, DeRose TJ, Rosen M, Evans J. Endoscopic harvest of fascia lata free flap in cadaveric model [Abstract]. J Neurol Surg B. 2012;73–A814. doi:10.1055/s-0032-1312232.
22. Gilles H. Experiences with fascia lata grafts in the operative treatment of facial paralysis. Proc R Soc Med. 1934;27:1372–82.
23. Flanagan JC, Campbell CB. The use of autogenous fascia lata to correct lid and orbital deformities. Trans Am Ophthalmol Soc. 1981;79:227–42.
24. Vlastou C. Facial paralysis. Microsurgery. 2005;26:278–87.
25. Chan DB, Temple HT, Latta LL, Mahure S, Dennis J, Kaplan LD. A biomechanical comparison of fan-folded, single-looped fascia lata with other graft tissues as a suitable substitute for anterior cruciate ligament reconstruction. Arthroscopy. 2010;26:1641–7.
26. Khiami F, Wajsfisz A, Meyer A, Rolland E, Catonné Y, Sariali E. Anterior cruciate ligament reconstruction with fascia lata using a minimally invasive arthroscopic harvesting technique. Orthop Traumatol Surg Res. 2013;99:99–105.
27. Culligan PJ, Murphy M, Blackwell L, Hammons G, Graham C, Heit MH. Long-term success of abdominal sacral colpopexy using synthetic mesh. Am J Obstet Gynecol. 2002;187:1473–82.
28. Tate SB, Blackwell L, Lorenz DJ, Steptoe MM, Culligan PJ. Randomized trial of fascia lata and polypropylene mesh for abdominal sacrocolpopexy: 5-year follow-up. Int Urogynecol J. 2011;22:137–43.
29. Corcos J, Schick E. The urinary sphincter. New York: Marcel Dekker; 2001.
30. Badlani GH, Davila GW, Michel MC, Rosette JJMCH. Continence. Current concepts and treatment strategies. London: Springer; 2009. ISBN 978-1-84628-510-3.
31. Rifaat MA, Gawad WS. The use of tensor fascia lata pedicled flap in reconstructing full thickness abdominal wall defects and groin defects following tumour ablation. J Egypt Natl Canc Inst. 2005;17:139–48.
32. Barron JN, Saad MN. Operative plastic and reconstructive surgery. Edinburgh: Churchill Livingstone; 1980.
33. Dubiel WT, Wigren A. Functional status of the lower extremity after resection of fascia lata. Acta Orthop Scand. 1974;45:599–613.
34. Iowa Head and Neck Protocols. Fascia lata harvest. University of Iowa Health Care. 2013. https://wiki.uiowa.edu/display/protocols/Fascia+Lata+Harvest. Accessed 5 Sept 2014.
35. Crawford JS. Repair of ptosis using frontalis muscle and fascia lata: a 20 year review. Ophthalmic Surg. 1977;8:31–40.
36. Wagner RS, Mauriello Jr JA, Nelson LB, Calhoun JH, Flanergan JC, Harley RD. Treatment of congenital ptosis with frontalis suspension: a comparison of suspensory materials. Ophthalmology. 1984;91:245–8.
37. Wilson ME, Johnson RW. Congenital ptosis, long term results of treatment using lyophilized fascia lata for frontalis suspensions. Ophthalmology. 1991;98:1234–7.

4 Axillary Endoscopic Breast Augmentation

José Maria Serra-Renom and José Maria Serra-Mestre

The use of the endoscopic axillary approach and the insertion of a cohesive, anatomically shaped silicone implant at a subfascial or submuscular level is our technique of choice for breast augmentation, provided that neither mastopexy nor glandular remodeling is required.

In our opinion, the axillary approach presents significant advantages over other alternatives. The use of endoscopy allows greater precision for controlling bleeding, creating the pocket, and detaching the pectoralis major muscle under direct vision. The scar is concealed in the highest fold of the armpit, not in the center of the breast, as it is with the periareolar approach, or in conspicuous sites, as it is if the access is via the inframammary fold (These scars are always visible in young patients, as a clear inframammary fold does not form until later). The axillary approach allows direct access to the subfascial or submuscular planes, respecting the integrity of the mammary parenchyma, the Cooper ligaments, and of course the axillary lymph nodes. As the skin of the armpit is fine and elastic, after making the incision as far as the subcutaneous plane, we can mobilize the skin above the outer edge of the pectoralis major muscle without reaching the axillary fat.

4.1 Surgical Technique

4.1.1 Implant Selection

To choose the implant required, we measure the distance from the midline to the anterior axillary line, which is the width, and the distance from the sternal notch to the nipple, which is the height. We then use a ruler to measure the projection of the breast, estimated from the central point of the inframammary fold to the intersection with a vertical line descending from the nipple areola complex. We also record the thickness of the adipose tissue, which we estimate using the pinching test at the level of the second rib [1–3].

In most cases, if the distance from the sternal notch to the nipple is less than 17 cm, we use a low high prosthesis. We use a moderate high prosthesis for distances between 17 and 21 cm, and a full high prosthesis for distances over 21 cm. As regards projection, if is less than 2 cm we choose a full projection implant; between 2 and 5 cm, we use one with moderate projection, and above 5 cm, one with low projection. We apply these guidelines for both round and anatomical prostheses.

4.1.2 Submuscular Dissection Technique

When the amount of breast tissue available to cover the implant is small (less than 2 cm according to the pinching test), the submuscular plane prevents the edge of the prosthesis from becoming evident in the upper quadrants of the breast. This is the case in about 75 % of the breast augmentations performed at our center. In addition, the use of an anatomical prosthesis allows satisfactory filling of the upper breast pole and provides sufficient volume and projection to the lower pole.

It is very important to place the patient correctly before starting surgery. The arms are extended and held in two arm boards at an angle of 90° at the level of the armpit. The gluteal region should coincide with the area where the table folds, so that the patient can be seated during the surgery without harming any anatomical structures.

Below we describe the sequence of the dissection, divided into areas [2]:

J.M. Serra-Renom, MD, PhD (✉) • J.M. Serra-Mestre, MD
Institute of Aesthetic and Plastic Surgery Dr. Serra Renom, Hospital Quiron, Barcelona Universitat, Internacional de Catalunya, Plaza Alfonso Comín, 5-7, Barcelona 08023, Spain
e-mail: serrarenom@gmail.com

E. Raposio (ed.), *Atlas of Endoscopic Plastic Surgery*, DOI 10.1007/978-3-319-19461-5_4

4.1.2.1 AREA I

First, an incision 4 cm long is made in the highest horizontal fold of the axilla (between the edge of the pectoralis major muscle at the front and the latissimus dorsi at the back). Then we continue the incision to a depth of 1 cm into the subcutaneous tissue (Fig. 4.1).

Maintaining the skin in tension, we make a subcutaneous dissection corresponding to the hairy area (if present) of about 5 cm long, preserving a thickness of about 1 cm (Fig. 4.2).

We perform the dissection this close to the surface so as not to affect the lymphatic drainage of the breast towards the armpit or damage the intercostobrachial nerve. After careful hemostasis, we mobilize the skin over the outer edge of the pectoral muscle (Fig. 4.3).

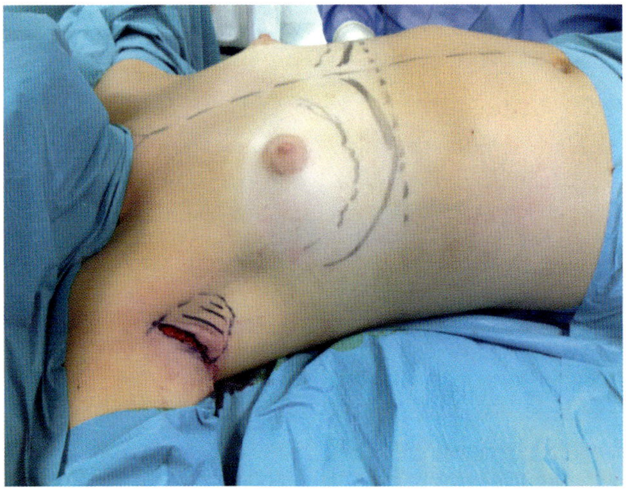

Fig. 4.1 Axillary incision

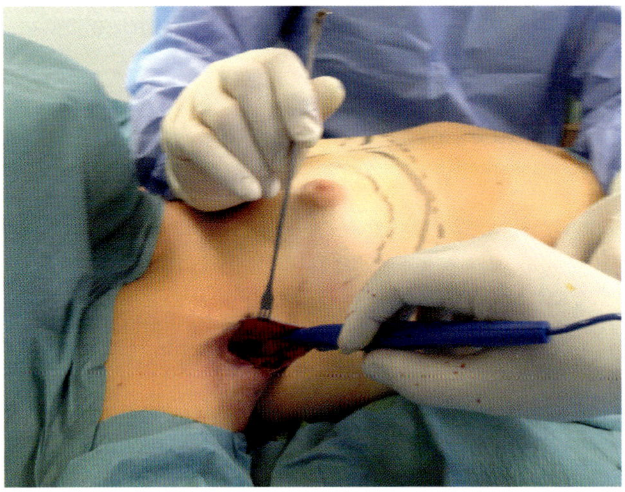

Fig. 4.2 Subcutaneous dissection corresponding to the hairy area (if present) of about 5 cm

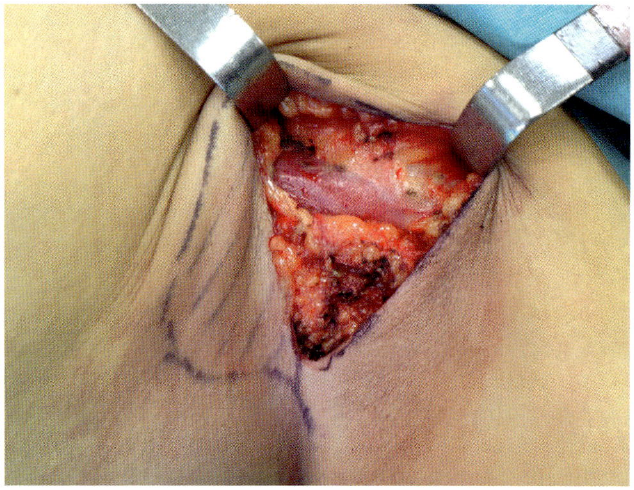

Fig. 4.3 Mobilization of the skin over the outer edge of the pectoral muscle

4.1.2.2 AREA II

With Metzenbaum scissors we open the plane between the pectoralis major and minor muscles (Fig. 4.4). It is important to follow the edge of the pectoralis major and to avoid going below the pectoralis minor; because of the pectoralis minor muscle's significant insertions in the third, fourth and fifth ribs, the bleeding will be much greater if this limit is surpassed.

4.1.2.3 AREA III

Next, we introduce the index finger beneath the pectoralis major muscle and make a blunt dissection, feeling the pectoralis major muscle above and the pectoralis minor below. If it is difficult to introduce the index finger, this means that we are below the pectoralis minor and we must start again.

We continue the digital blunt dissection towards the fourth rib, stopping when the muscle attachment is palpable (Fig. 4.5).

We never perform muscle detachment in a blunt manner. We then place gauzes with warm saline solution, and create the same submuscular pocket on the contralateral side.

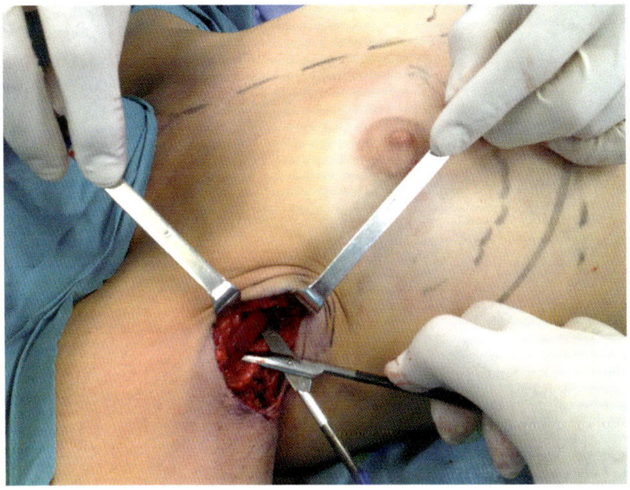

Fig. 4.4 Opening of the plane between the pectoralis major and minor muscles

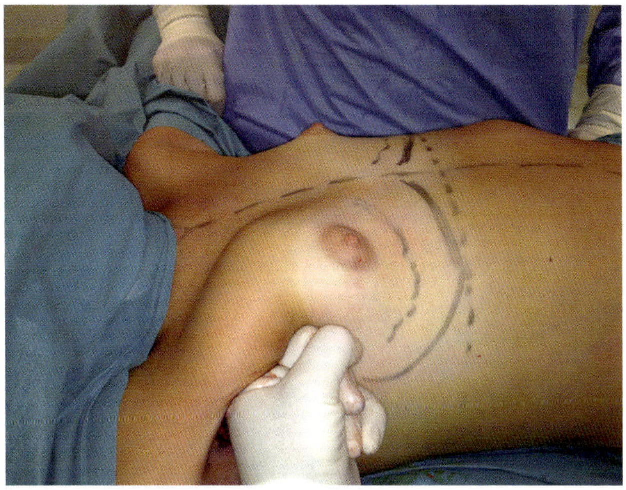

Fig. 4.5 Blunt dissection towards the fourth rib

4.1.2.4 AREA IV

We insert the Serra-Renom [4] endoscopic retractor (Snowden-Pencer; Tucker, GA, USA) with a 10-mm 0° telescope, and we use the coagulation and suction endoscalpel to detach the pectoralis major muscle at the fourth, fifth, and sixth ribs (Fig. 4.6).

When we reach the sixth rib, the muscle fibers are tense because we maintain the retractor angled upwards (Fig. 4.7).

We are therefore able to section them confidently. We stop when we see the fat, so as not to injure the skin (Fig. 4.8).

This section of the muscle fibers of the pectoralis major muscle at the sixth rib runs from the axillary line to within 1.5 cm from the sternal border. At the level of the medial insertions of the pectoralis major muscle, we never dissect above the fourth rib, so as not to section the perforating branches of the internal mammary artery and to avoid the risk of symmastia.

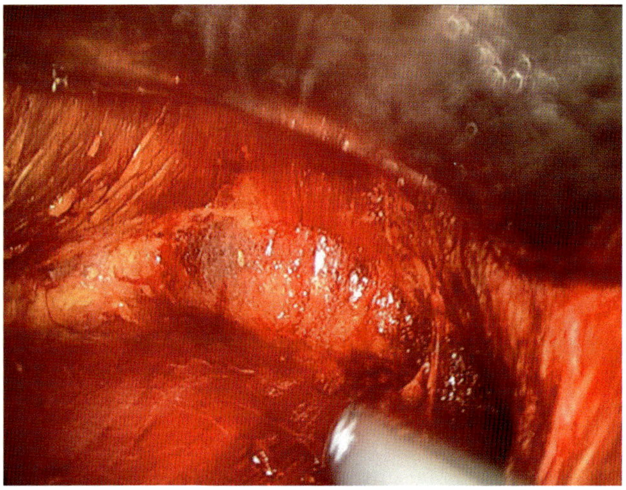

Fig. 4.6 Endoscopic dissection as far as the costal insertions of the pectoralis major

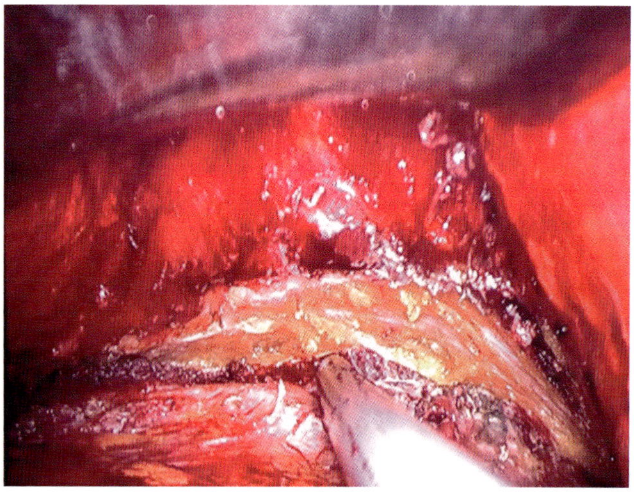

Fig. 4.8 Finalization of dissection on observing the subcutaneous fat, so as not to damage the skin

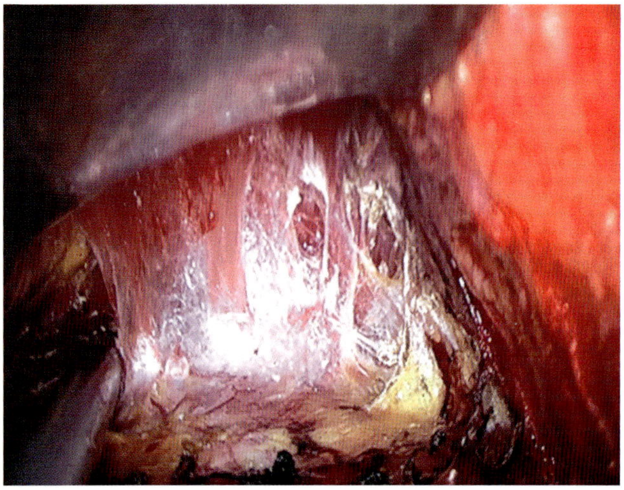

Fig. 4.7 Detachment of the pectoral muscle from its costal insertions

4.1.2.5 AREA V

In practically all breast augmentations, it is necessary to move the inframammary fold downward. We do this using blunt dissection with the Digman dissector under endoscopic view. As this area may bleed, we then perform hemostasis using the endoscopic scalpel if necessary.

4.1.2.6 AREA VI

This area extends from the lateral edge of the pectoralis major muscle to the anterior axillary line and the outer lower quadrant. It is very important not to perform dissection with electrocautery, because this process may damage the sensory nerves that innervate the nipple areola complex; therefore, blunt dissection is performed using the Digman dissector under direct and endoscopic vision (Fig. 4.9). We then perform rigorous hemostasis.

After creating the pocket as described above, we now insert the sizers. The sizers tell us whether the expectations of the patient can be met, which prosthesis is the best for the particular patient, and whether the two pockets are the same or if some minor retouches are required to achieve symmetry before inserting the final implant. The sizer on one side corresponds to the width of the patient; on the other, the dimensions of the sizer we insert depend on the patient's expectations, as discussed during the preoperative interview.

We then insert the definitive implant and check that it is correctly positioned by endoscopic visualization of landmarks in the posterior part of the prosthesis (Figs. 4.10 and 4.11).

We close the skin with subcutaneous stitches and an intradermal suture. We place a moldable dressing, clearly marking the fold and the upper poles; with micropore tapes, we correctly define the intermammary cleft.

It is very important that the patient should sleep in the supine position for the first 2 weeks of the postoperative period. The patient is seen after 7 days, at which time the bandage is removed and a Velcro band is placed at the level of the second rib.

Figure 4.12 illustrates a clinical case of breast augmentation via the submuscular axillary approach.

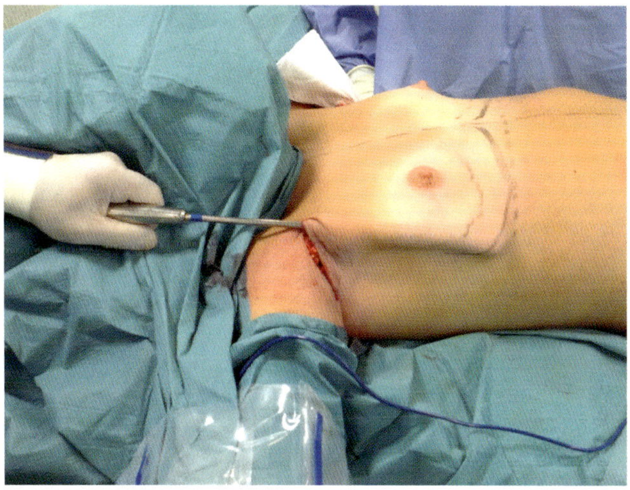

Fig. 4.9 Downward displacement of the inframammary fold and lateral extension of the pocket with the Digman dissector

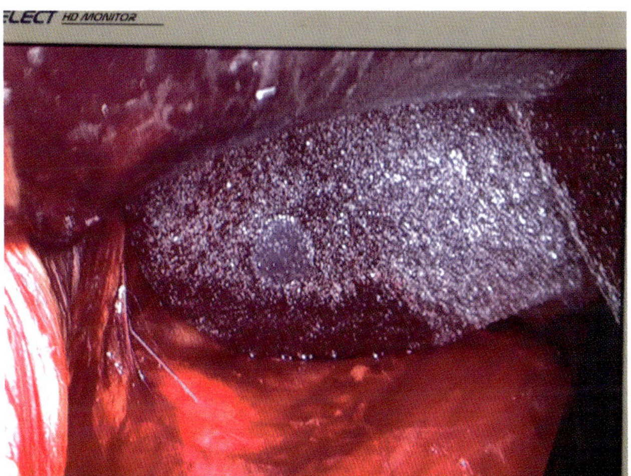

Fig. 4.10 Endoscopic visualization of landmarks in the posterior part of the prosthesis

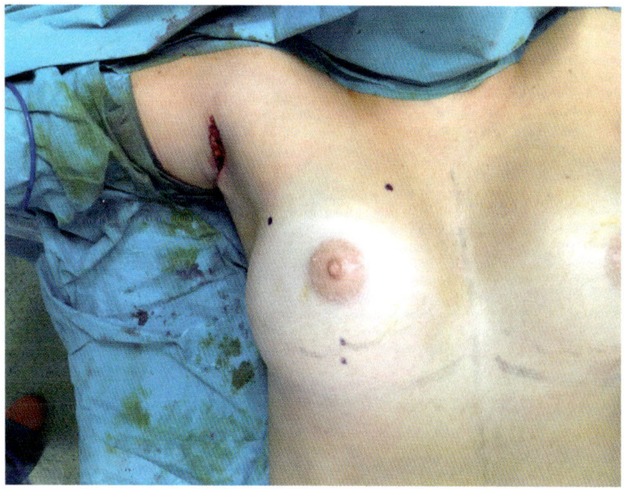

Fig. 4.11 Checking and marking of the position of the landmarks in the prosthesis

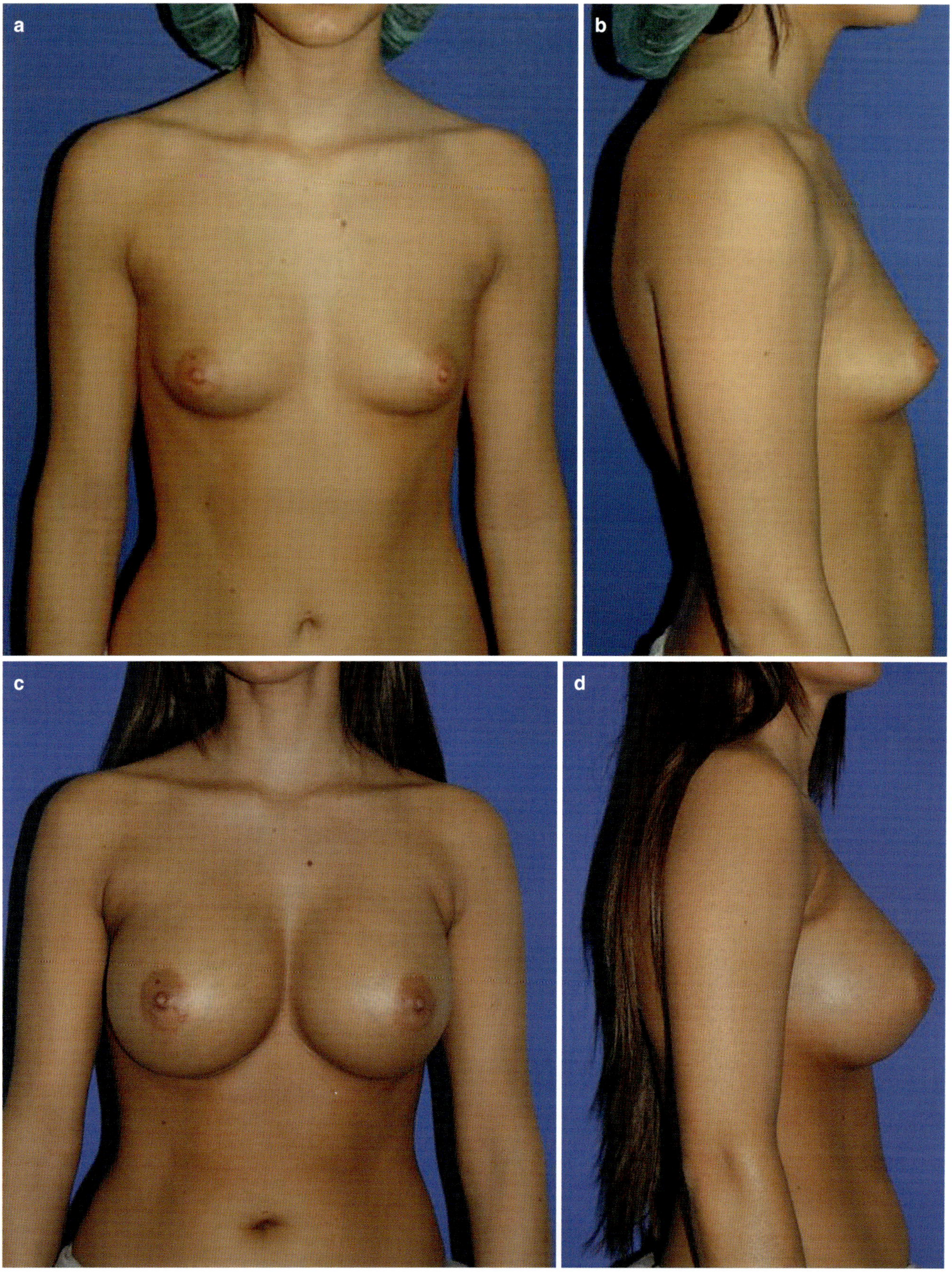

Fig. 4.12 Clinical case 1. Breast augmentation via submuscular axillary approach. (**a**), Frontal preoperative image. (**b**), Preoperative profile. (**c**), Frontal postoperative image. (**d**), Postoperative profile

4.1.3 Subfascial Dissection Technique

We perform subfascial dissection in patients with abundant adipose tissue (more than 2 cm on the pinching test) who do not require large increases, and in professional athletes (tennis players, climbers, and so on) who do not want to alter the pectoralis major muscle in any way. We have limited the indications considerably because the edge of the prosthesis in thin women with small breasts is highly visible in the outer upper and lower quadrants. There is also a risk of symmastia in the long term, though it is rare.

The placement of the patient, the marking of the incision, and the subcutaneous dissection are all the same as for the submuscular approach (Figs. 4.13 and 4.14).

After reaching the lateral border of the pectoralis major muscle, we make an incision in the fascia (Fig. 4.15) and perform dissection on the muscle fibers and below the fascia of the pectoralis major muscle (Fig. 4.16), using the Serra-Renom endoscopic retractor (Snowden-Pencer, Tucker, GA, USA) with a 10-mm 0° telescope [4].

The dissection of the muscle must be as atraumatic as possible to avoid tearing the muscle fibers and to maintain the integrity of the fascia (Fig. 4.17).

It is important to perform careful hemostasis throughout the dissection process.

On reaching the distal limit, the fascia is incised horizontally with the endoscalpel at the level of the sixth rib, so it is already separated from the muscle. We then perform subcutaneous dissection down to the point where the new inframammary fold will be created. This dissection is carried out in a blunt manner so as not to injure the skin.

It is very important when making the pocket not to go further than 1.5 cm from the sternal midline, because of the risk of symmastia. At the lateral level, after passing the edge of the full extent of the pectoralis major muscle, we perform blunt dissection around the side pocket to avoid damaging the nerves that provide sensation to the nipple-areola complex. After creating this pocket on either side, we perform rigorous hemostasis, which we verify by endoscopy. After using the sizers, we insert the definitive prostheses (Fig. 4.18), and check by endoscopy that the landmarks in the posterior wall of the implant are correctly positioned (Fig. 4.19).

We then introduce a suction drain and close the skin with subcutaneous stitches and an intradermal suture. We attach a moldable dressing, clearly marking the inframammary fold, the upper pole, and the midline to strengthen the intermammary cleft [5–7].

Figure 4.20 illustrates a clinical case of breast augmentation via the submuscular axillary approach.

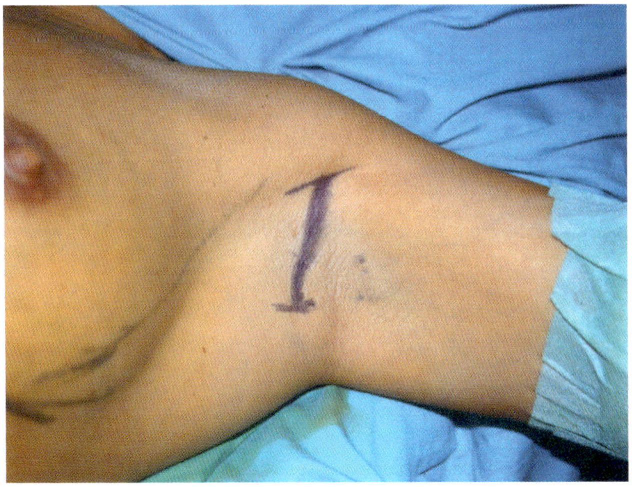

Fig. 4.13 Axillary incision

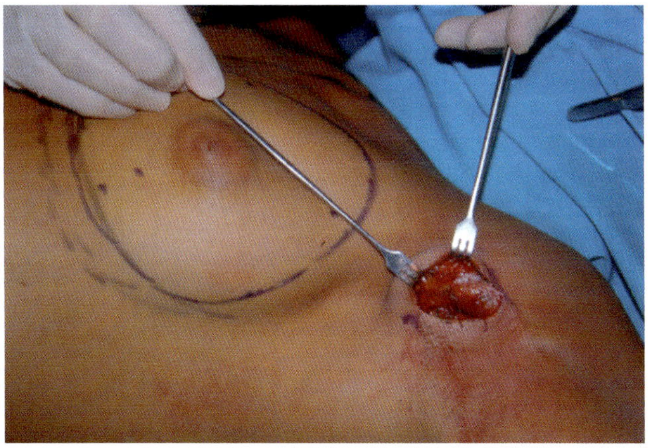

Fig. 4.14 Mobilization of the skin over the outer edge of the pectoral muscle

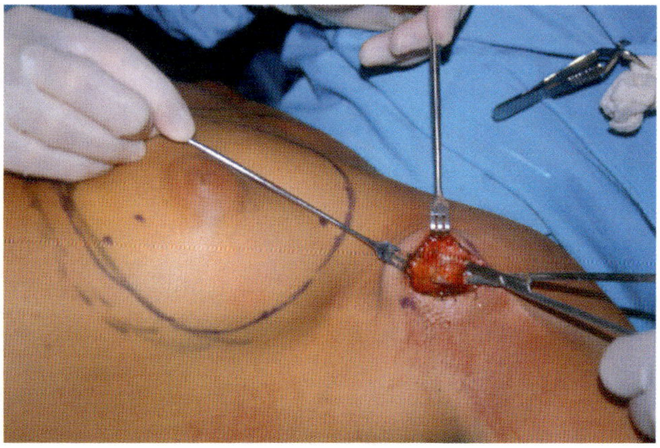

Fig. 4.15 Incision in the fascia

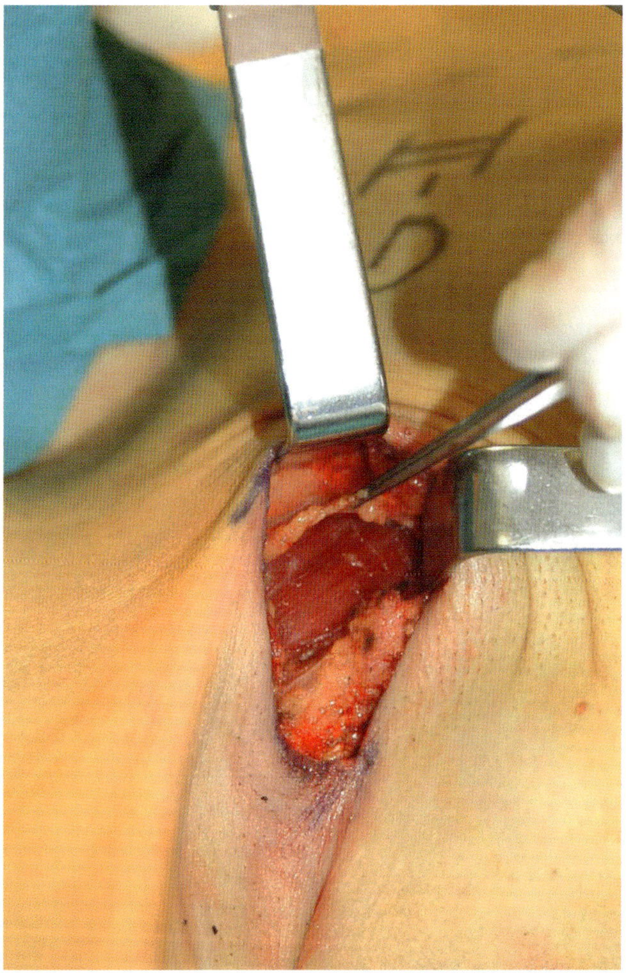

Fig. 4.16 Subfascial dissection

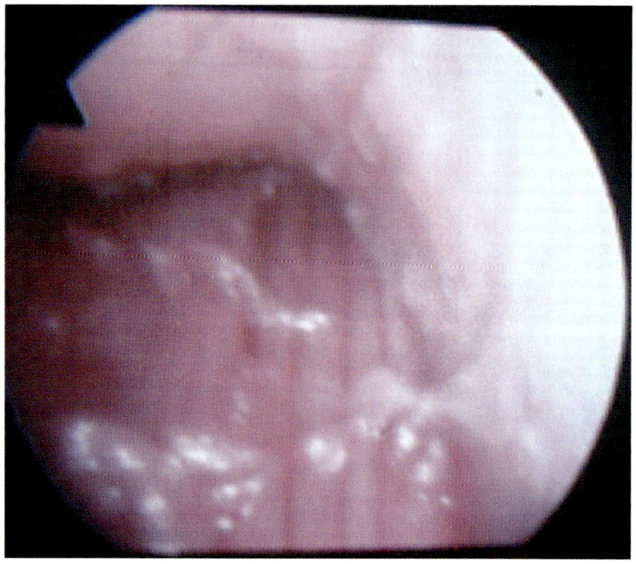

Fig. 4.17 Endoscopic subfascial dissection

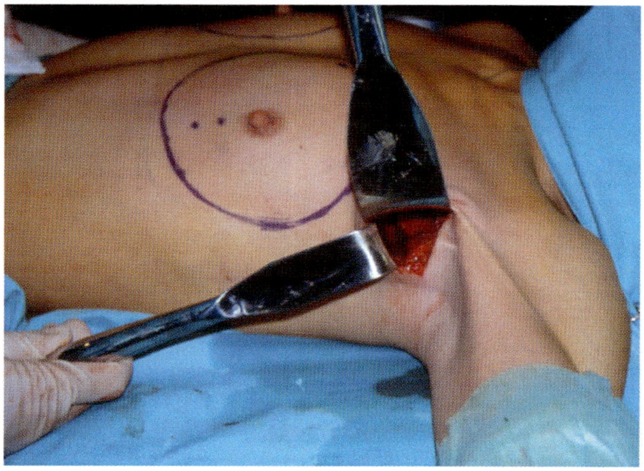

Fig. 4.18 Introduction of the implant

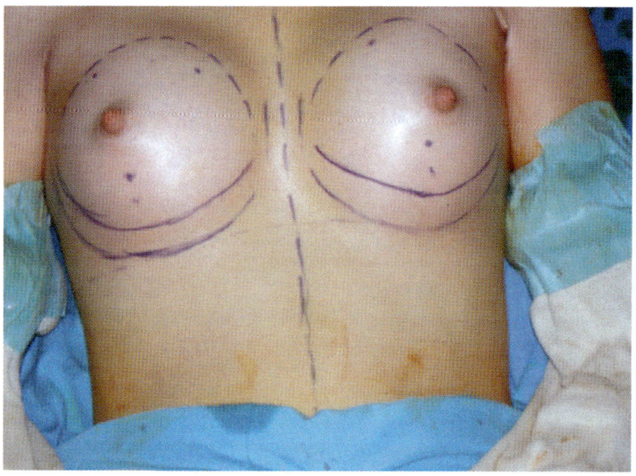

Fig. 4.19 Checking and marking of the position of the landmarks in the prosthesis

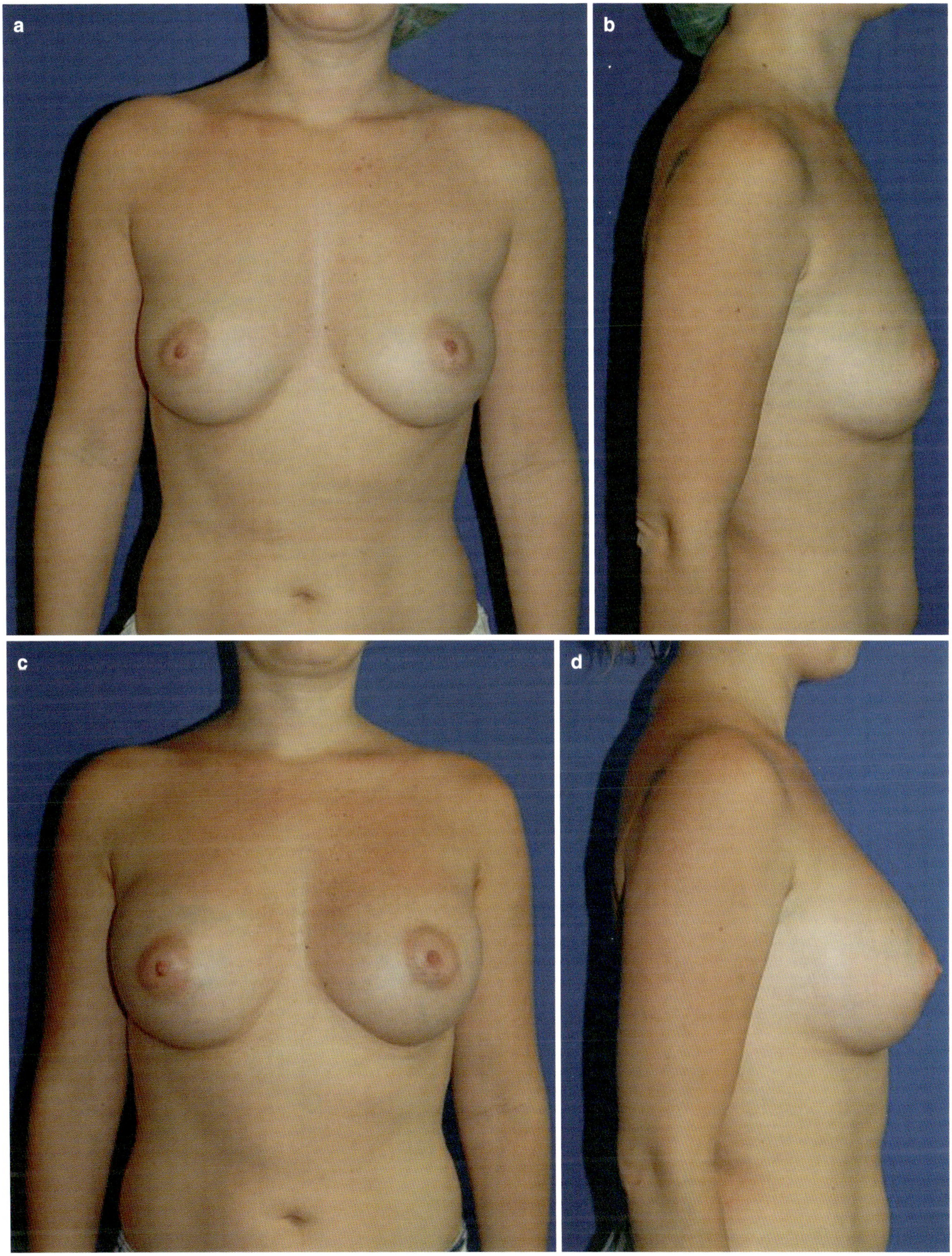

Fig. 4.20 Clinical case 2. Breast augmentation via subfascial axillary approach. (**a**), Frontal preoperative image. (**b**), Preoperative profile. (**c**), Frontal postoperative image. (**d**), Postoperative profile

4.1.4 Mammoplasty for Tuberous Breasts (Grade I–II)

For these cases of mild or moderate tuberosity (grades I–II, according to Grolleau's classification) our paper published in *Aesthetic Plastic Surgery* [8] described a new technique of breast augmentation via a transaxillary approach using endoscopy and radial cuts for expansion of the lower poles. This technique also applies an axillary subfascial approach as far as the new inframammary fold, as described above.

We use sizers to check for the double bubble. After choosing the right sizer, if a double bubble is present, we mark the area with a felt pen and remove the sizer. Then, at the site of the old inframammary fold we section the fascia and constrictor ring, making cuts 1 cm deep, both vertically (to achieve expansion in width) and horizontally (to achieve expansion in height) (Fig. 4.21).

The choice of prosthesis depends on the preferences of the patient, the need to correct the double bubble, and the adaptation of the glandular tissue. We stress the importance of inserting an anatomical prosthesis with moderate or high projection to obtain volume in the lower quadrants.

If a slight double bubble persists after the placement of the final prosthesis, subcutaneous fat grafting at the level of the double bubble is particularly useful (Fig. 4.22).

In this way we obtain satisfactory breast augmentation with correction of grade I–II tuberosity, and the scar is concealed in the highest horizontal fold of the axilla. It is important to note that these patients with tuberous breasts grade I and II are not previously aware of any alteration; they only want breast augmentation, and it is very important not to have to create scars or perform radical surgery in order to change the shape of the breast.

Figure 4.23 illustrates a clinical case of breast augmentation via the axillary approach in a patient with tuberous breasts.

The approach described here cannot be used for grade III tuberous breasts, however. Open remodeling surgery is required for these patients [9].

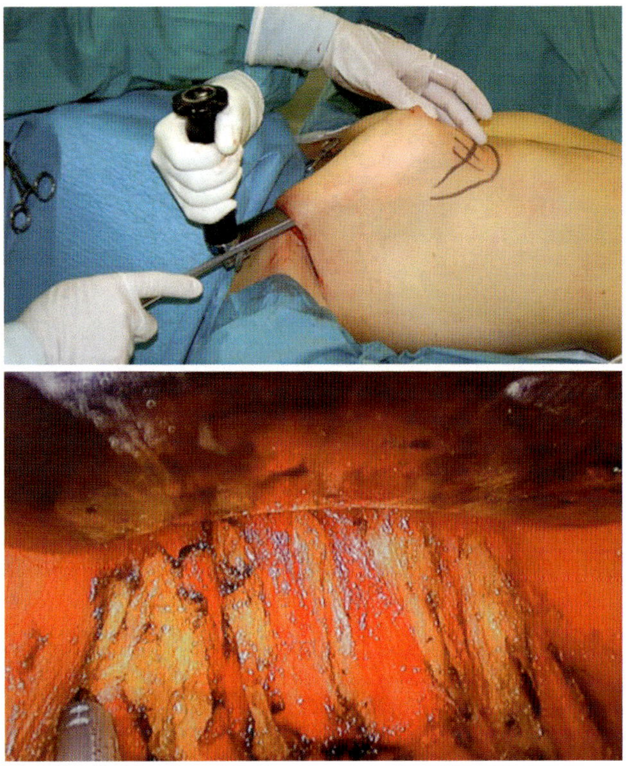

Fig. 4.21 Horizontal and vertical sections to expand the mammary tissue in a patient with tuberous breasts

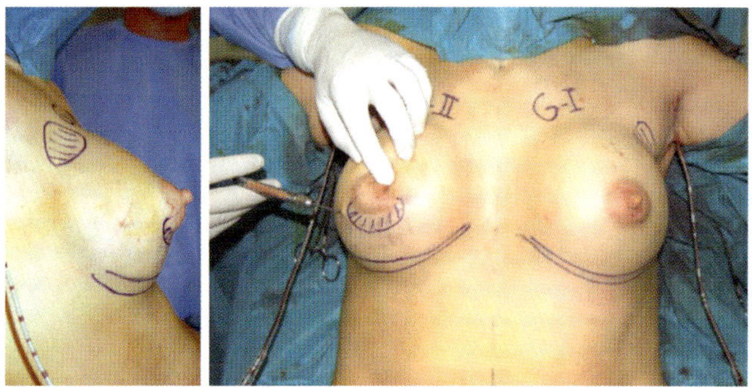

Fig. 4.22 Fat grafting at the level of the double bubble, if it persists

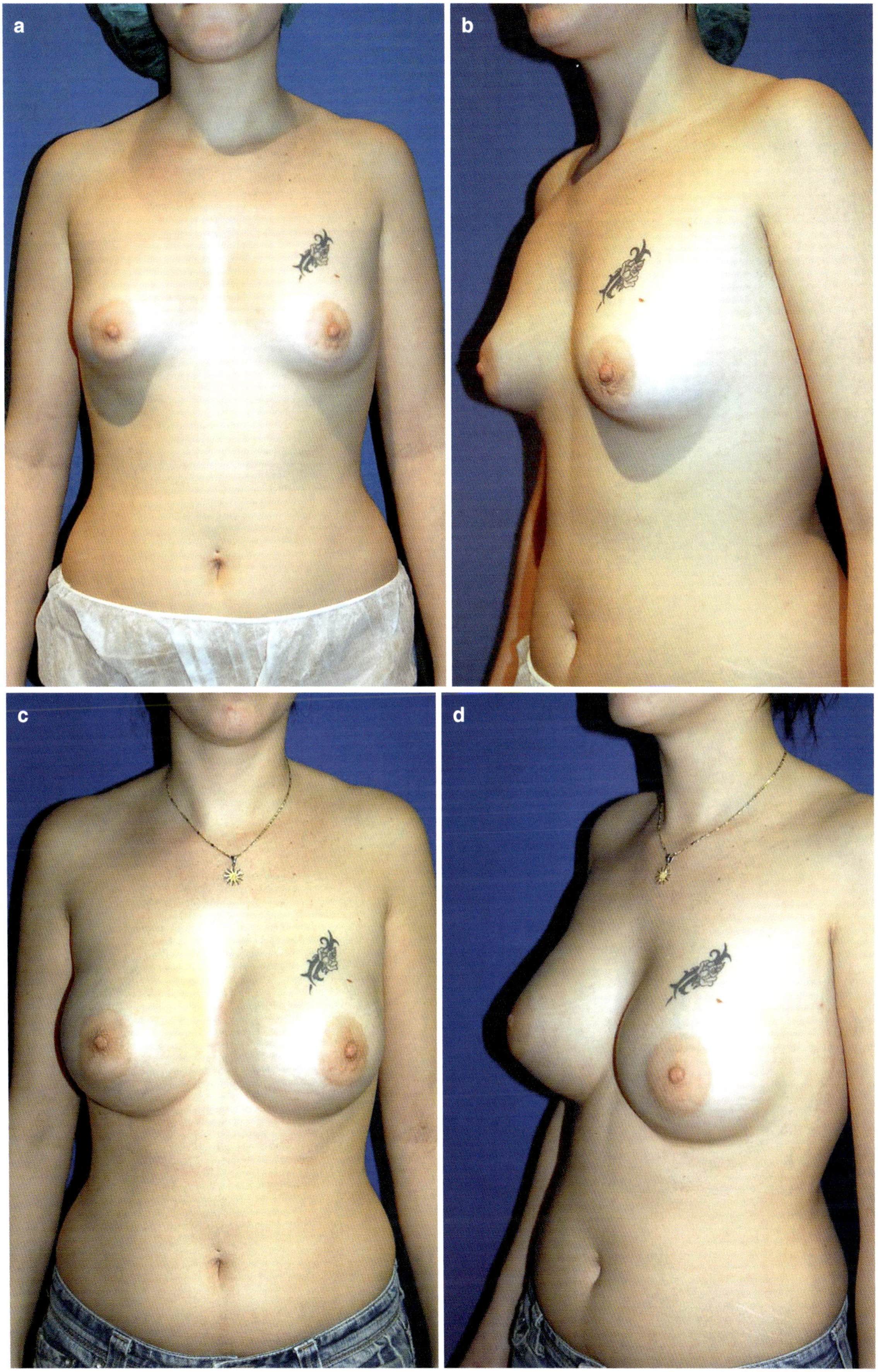

Fig. 4.23 Clinical case 3. Breast augmentation via axillary approach in tuberous breasts. (**a**), Frontal preoperative image. (**b**), Preoperative oblique view. (**c**), Frontal postoperative image. (**d**), Postoperative oblique view

Conclusions

Our protocol for breast augmentation with anatomical prostheses via an endoscopic axillary approach (either subfascial or submuscular) achieves highly satisfactory results. Great accuracy is required in the assessment of breast shape, height, projection, pinching test, width, and placement of the new fold in order to select the appropriate prosthesis and obtain good results. Sizers are very useful to guide the choice of prosthesis. As a result, we obtain a satisfactory breast augmentation with cohesive, anatomically shaped prostheses and excellent postoperative outcome. While respecting the integrity, lactation, and functionality of the mammary gland and without any alterations in the sensitivity of the nipple areola complex, we are able to reestablish a harmonious body image for the patient.

References

1. Tebbetts JB. A system for breast implant selection based on patient tissue characteristics and implant-soft tissue dynamics. Plast Reconstr Surg. 2002;109:1396–409.
2. Serra-Renom JM, Serra-Mestre JM. Mamoplastia de aumento con ubicación de implante retromuscular. In: Berrocal M, editor. Las cuatro estaciones de las mamas. Colombia: Editorial Impresión Médica; 2014. p. 253–70.
3. Serra Renom JM, Vila R. Endoscopia en cirugía plástica y estética. Barcelona: Ed Masson S.A; 1995.
4. Serra Renom JM. Retractor with mobile endoscope. Plast Reconstr Surg. 1997;100:529–31.
5. Graf RM, Bernardes A, Rippel R, Araujo LR, Damasio RC, Auersvald A. Subfascial breast implant: a new procedure. Plast Reconstr Surg. 2003;111:904–8.
6. Serra Renom JM, Fernandez Garrido M, Yoon T. Augmentation mammaplasty with anatomic soft, cohesive silicone implant using the transaxillary approach at a subfascial level with endoscopic assistance. Plast Reconstr Surg. 2005;116:640–5.
7. Serra Renom JM, Muñoz del Olmo J. Aumento mamario con colocación de prótesis anatómicas por vía axilar a nivel subfascial mediante ayuda endoscópica. Cirugía Estética Plástica. 2008;7:22–6.
8. Serra-Renom JM, Muñoz-Olmo J, Serra-Mestre JM. Endoscopic-assisted aesthetic augmentation of tuberous breasts and fat grafting to correct the double bubble. Aesthetic Plast Surg. 2012;36:1114–9.
9. Serra Renom JM, Muñoz-Olmo J, Serra Mestre JM. Treatment of grade 3 tuberous breasts with Puckett's tecnique (modified) and fat grafting to correct the constricting ring. Aesthetic Plast Surg. 2011;35:773–81.

5 Transaxillary Endoscopic Subfascial Breast Augmentation

Joseph P. Hunstad and Nicholas A. Flugstad

Transaxillary endoscopic breast augmentation (in the submuscular pocket) was described by Price et al. in 1994 [1]. Compared with previously described blind transaxillary approaches, the transaxillary endoscopic approach maintains the advantage of inconspicuous scars and in addition affords direct vision for excellent control of the pocket dissection [2]. The endoscopic camera also allows a magnified image of the dissection plane. The procedure does require additional equipment, setup, and possibly operative time compared with the two most popular non-endoscopic approaches, inframammary and periareolar incisions.

With the transaxillary endoscopic approach, saline or silicone gel implants may be used. Transaxillary endoscopic breast augmentation can be performed with implant placement above or below the pectoralis major muscle. Graf et al. [3, 4] introduced breast augmentation in the subfascial plane via the transaxillary approach in 2000. The subfascial technique, in which the implant is placed in a pocket beneath the pectoralis major fascia and above the muscle fibers, offers potential advantages over submuscular placement that include less animation deformity and possibly less displacement of the implant over time [5–7]. Compared with subglandular placement, subfascial placement may offer a thin but substantial additional layer of coverage to minimize implant visibility [8].

J.P. Hunstad, MD, FACS
The Hunstad Kortesis Center for Cosmetic Plastic Surgery, Huntersville, NC, USA

Division of Plastic Surgery, The University of North Carolina, Chapel Hill, NC, USA

Plastic Surgery Division, Department of Surgery, Carolinas Medical Ctr., University Hospital, Charlotte, NC, USA
e-mail: jphunstad@gmail.com

N.A. Flugstad, MD (✉)
The Hunstad Kortesis Center for Cosmetic Plastic Surgery, 12800 Statesville Road, Huntersville, NC 28078, USA
e-mail: nick.flugstad@gmail.com

E. Raposio (ed.), *Atlas of Endoscopic Plastic Surgery*, DOI 10.1007/978-3-319-19461-5_5

5.1 Surgical Technique

5.1.1 Setup

The required instruments are pictured in Fig. 5.1.

Endoscopic instruments include a 10-mm, 30° angled endoscope, endoscopic cautery and suction, Deaver retractor, strong curved Mayo scissors, and several blunt dissectors. An endoscopic tower with high-resolution video monitor and adequate operating room space are required. The patient is under general anesthesia, positioned supine with her arms out at 90°. The endoscopic tower is set up at the foot of the operating table for ease of viewing when dissecting on the left and right sides. Prep and drape are done in the usual fashion, with the axillary area fully exposed.

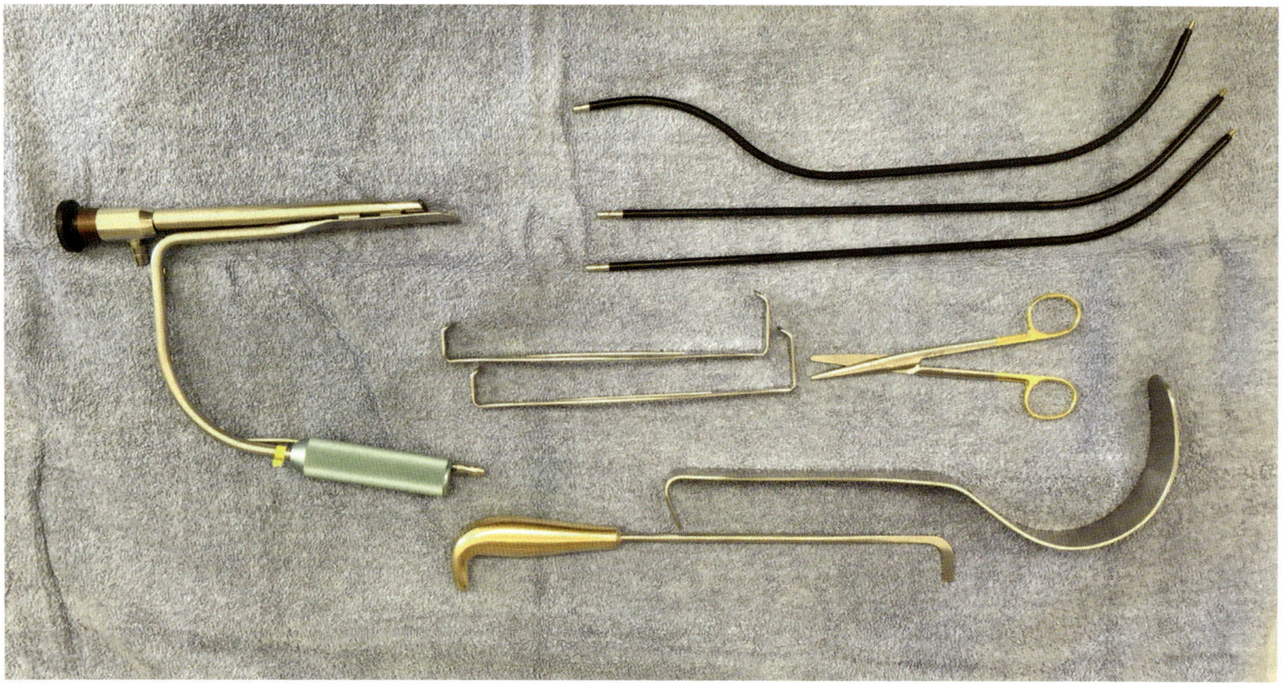

Fig. 5.1 The typical instrumentation required for endoscopic subfascial breast augmentation. On the left is pictured the 30°, 10-mm endoscope with retractor

5.1.2 Patient Markings

The patient is marked in a standing position. The anterior border of the axillary fold is marked (Fig. 5.2), ensuring that the incision is placed posterior to this point. The incision is marked in an AP direction, in the apex of the axilla (Figs. 5.3 and 5.4). The anterior end of the incision must be 1–2 cm from the axillary fold to prevent visibility. The midline is marked with a vertical line, and the inframammary fold and the outline of the planned dissection are then marked (Fig. 5.5).

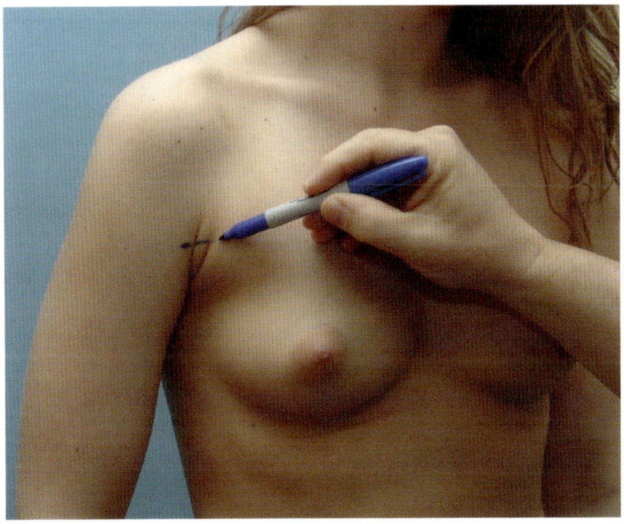

Fig. 5.2 First, the anterior border of the axillary fold is marked with the patient standing with her arms at rest. The incision should never extend anterior to this line

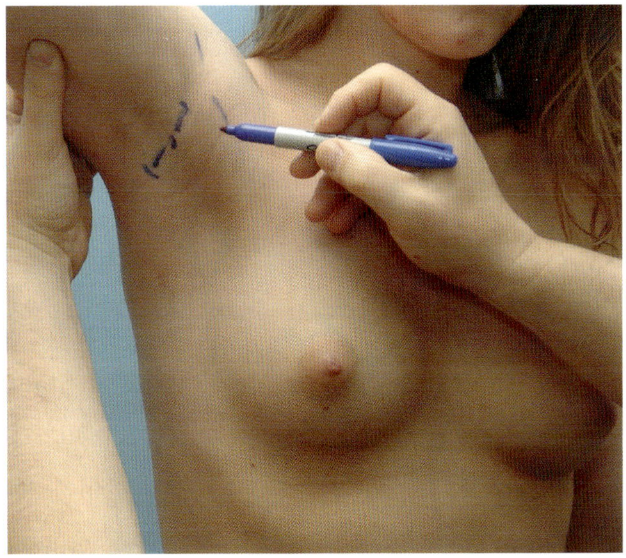

Fig. 5.4 The planned incision is shown. It is 1–2 cm posterior to the anterior axillary fold to ensure invisibility with the arms in repose. An incision 4–5 cm in length is designed

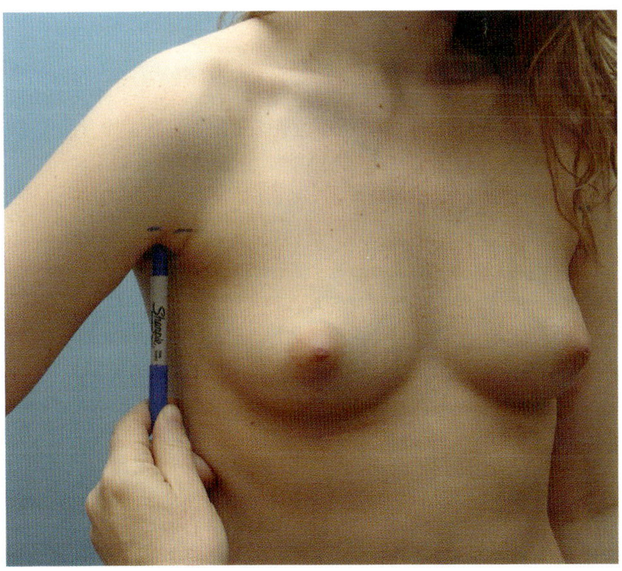

Fig. 5.3 The axillary apex is marked in the highest part of the armpit. This is done with the patient placing her hand on her hip and flexing her pectoralis major muscle

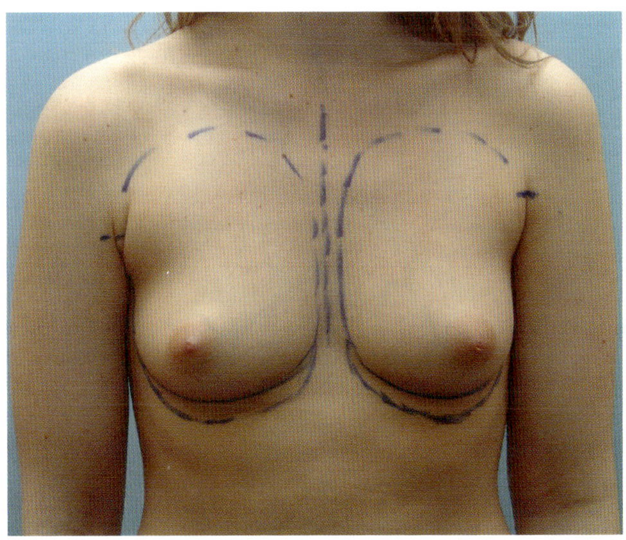

Fig. 5.5 The planned outline of dissection. This patient's inframammary fold will be lowered. The incisions are invisible in this position

5.1.3 Procedure

A 2-0 nylon figure-of-eight suture is placed at the anterior end of the marked incision. This prevents skin tearing and inadvertent extension of the incision anteriorly during retraction and implant placement. The incision is made and the subcutaneous space is opened (Figs. 5.6, 5.7, and 5.8).

Curved Mayo scissors are used to spread the soft tissues until the pectoralis major fascia is visualized (Fig. 5.9).

Spreading in this portion while exposing the muscle helps to preserve sensory nerves such as the intercostobrachial nerve [9]. For this reason, it is important to avoid posterior dissection within the axillary fat [10]. Once the pectoralis major fascia is exposed, the fascia is opened the muscle fibers are exposed. The endoscope is introduced (Fig. 5.10), and the subfascial plane is developed.

The subfascial plane is best dissected using firm traction with the retractor and electrocautery to release the fascia from the muscle (Fig. 5.11). The subfascial plane is not easily dissected bluntly, but we do reserve blunt dissection to adjust the pocket and lower the inframammary fold, if necessary.

Hemostasis must be performed prospectively as dissection is done. The pocket is dissected superiorly, then laterally and inferiorly (Fig. 5.12).

After precise pocket dissection, an inflatable or silicone gel tester implant is placed (Fig. 5.13).

The patient is sat up and any areas of further dissection are marked and addressed with endoscope and cautery. With the patient sitting up, blunt dissection is used to perform any final pocket refinements. Meticulous hemostasis must be ensured, as any ongoing bleeding may be difficult to identify in the endoscopic approach. The permanent implant is placed, manually or with a Keller Funnel (Keller Medical; Stuart, FL). The surgeon must ensure that the implant is fully seated in the pocket. Vicryl sutures are used to close the pectoralis fascia, preventing axillary displacement, and to close the subcutaneous layer. Finally, skin closure is performed with absorbable monofilament suture.

5.1.4 Postoperative Care

A surgical bra and bandeau are typically applied. The bandeau may prevent the implants from being displaced cephalad in the postoperative period. We initiate range of motion exercises of the arms and shoulders in the immediate postoperative period. Lifting restrictions are maintained for 4 weeks. Paper tape is placed on the incisions and replaced weekly for 2–3 weeks.

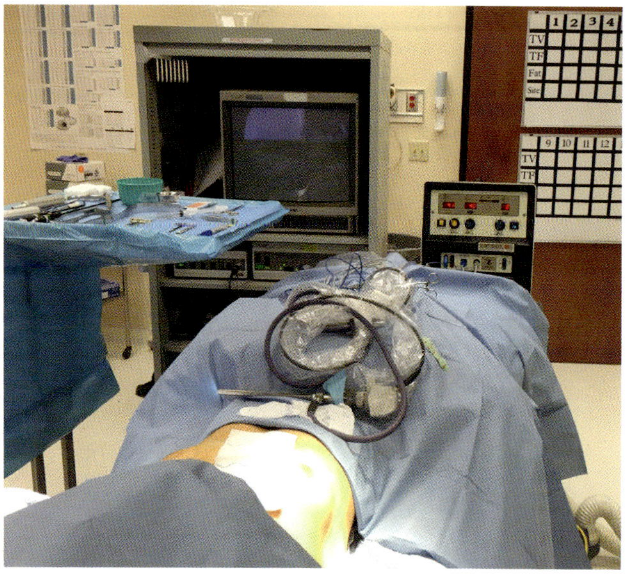

Fig. 5.6 The patient is positioned supine with the arms out at 90°. The endoscopic tower is set up at the patient's feet for ease of viewing during dissection on each side. Care is taken to ensure that all equipment is properly secured and can be operated while standing on the right or left side

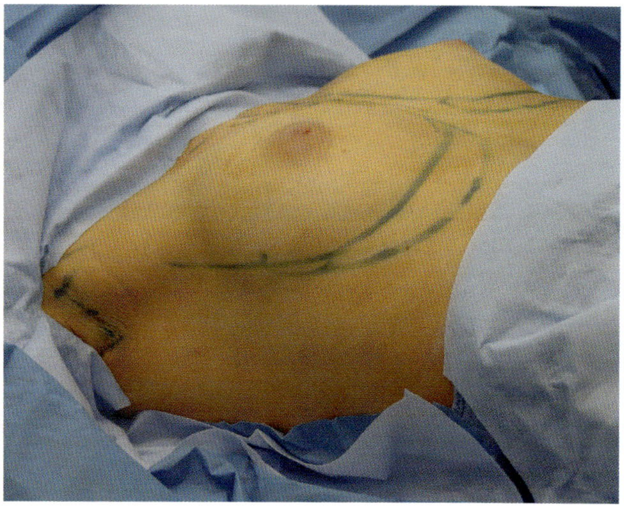

Fig. 5.7 The patient is positioned on the operating table with the arms out at 90°. The planned incision and area of dissection are shown

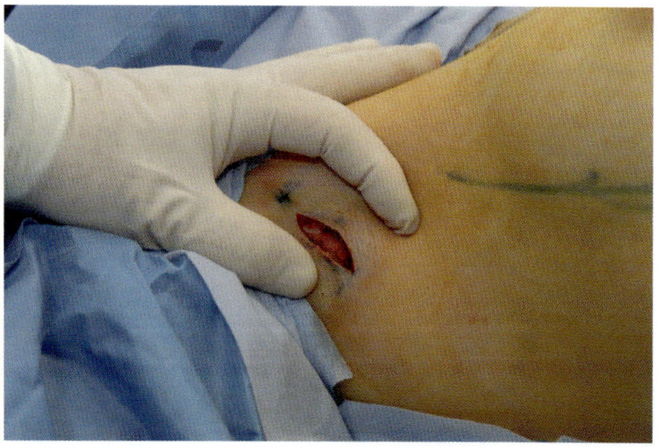

Fig. 5.8 The incision is made and the subcutaneous layer is opened with electrocautery

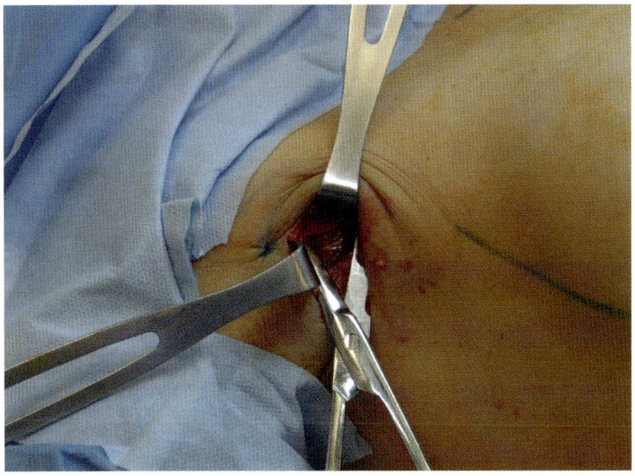

Fig. 5.9 Spreading with a curved Mayo scissors is done to identify the fascia of the pectoralis major muscle

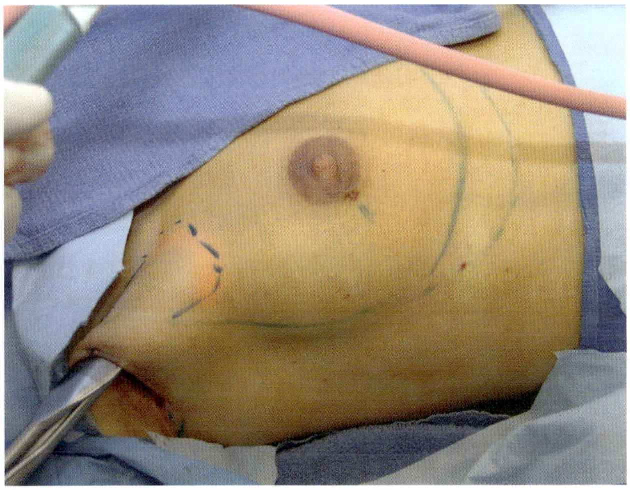

Fig. 5.10 With the space opened, the endoscope is introduced. The room is darkened to enhance visualization. The table height is adjusted to ensure a proper working position for the surgeon

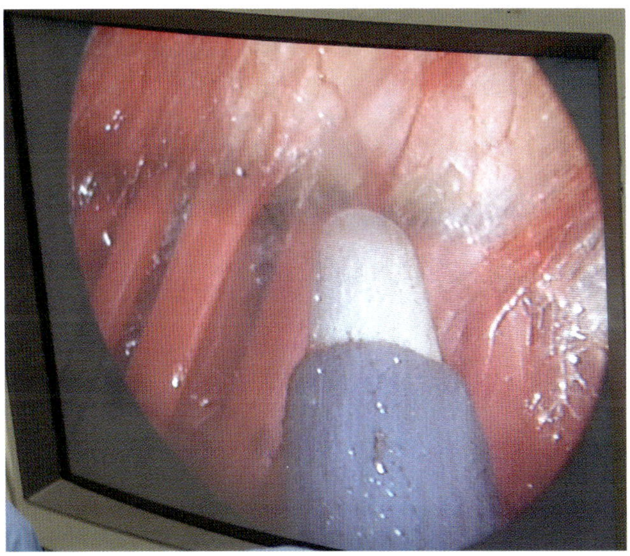

Fig. 5.11 The electrocautery is used to elevate the subfascial plane. Firm retraction is required to develop this plane. The plane is very distinct

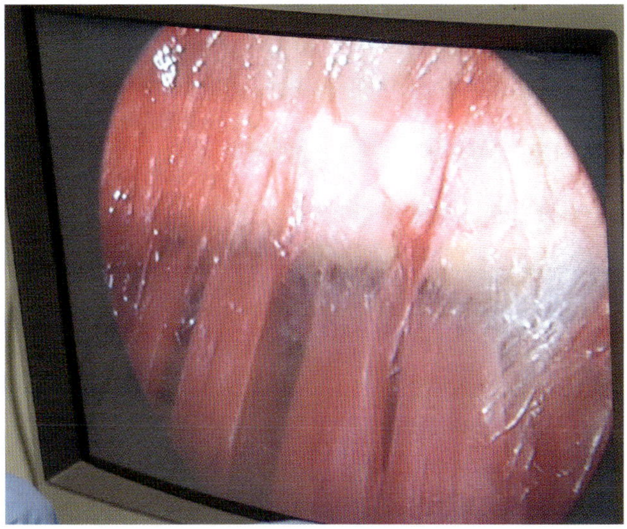

Fig. 5.12 View of the subfascial plane elevated; the pectoralis major fibers are seen in the lower half of the picture

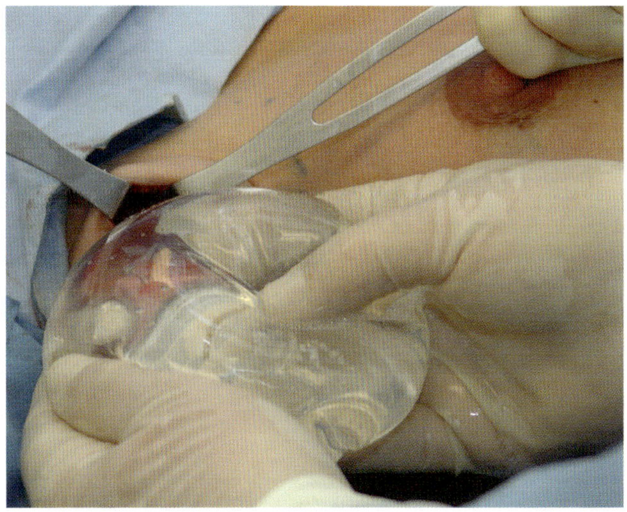

Fig. 5.13 The pocket is irrigated and the retractors are positioned. Sizers are placed and the patient is sat up to verify the pocket dissection. Finally, the permanent implant is placed manually in the pocket

5.2 Complications

Complications, such has infection, hematoma, and implant malposition are similar to those occurring with other approaches. It should be kept in mind that if a postoperative hematoma does occur, it may be difficult to view and control the bleeding endoscopically. In such a situation, the surgeon should have a low threshold for the use of an inframammary incision. Although unusual, most pocket revision surgery requires an inframammary approach. Some revision surgery, such as minor capsulotomy, capsulorrhaphy, or change of implant due to size preference can be safely performed endoscopically [11].

Conclusions

In our experience, endoscopic subfascial transaxillary breast augmentation is associated with natural, lasting results and high patient satisfaction (Figs. 5.14, 5.15, and 5.16).

Compared with traditional, non-endoscopic transaxillary methods, blind dissection and associated increased bleeding are minimized [10]. We offer subfascial placement to patients who have adequate breast tissue for implant coverage (typically >2 cm pinch test in the upper pole), ensuring that the superior edge of the implant will not be palpable. If the upper pole breast tissue is inadequate, a submuscular pocket should be considered. The endoscopic transaxillary approach is not practical for major revision surgery such as pocket change or total capsulectomy. Patients desiring primary breast augmentation who wish to avoid a scar on their breast may choose this procedure.

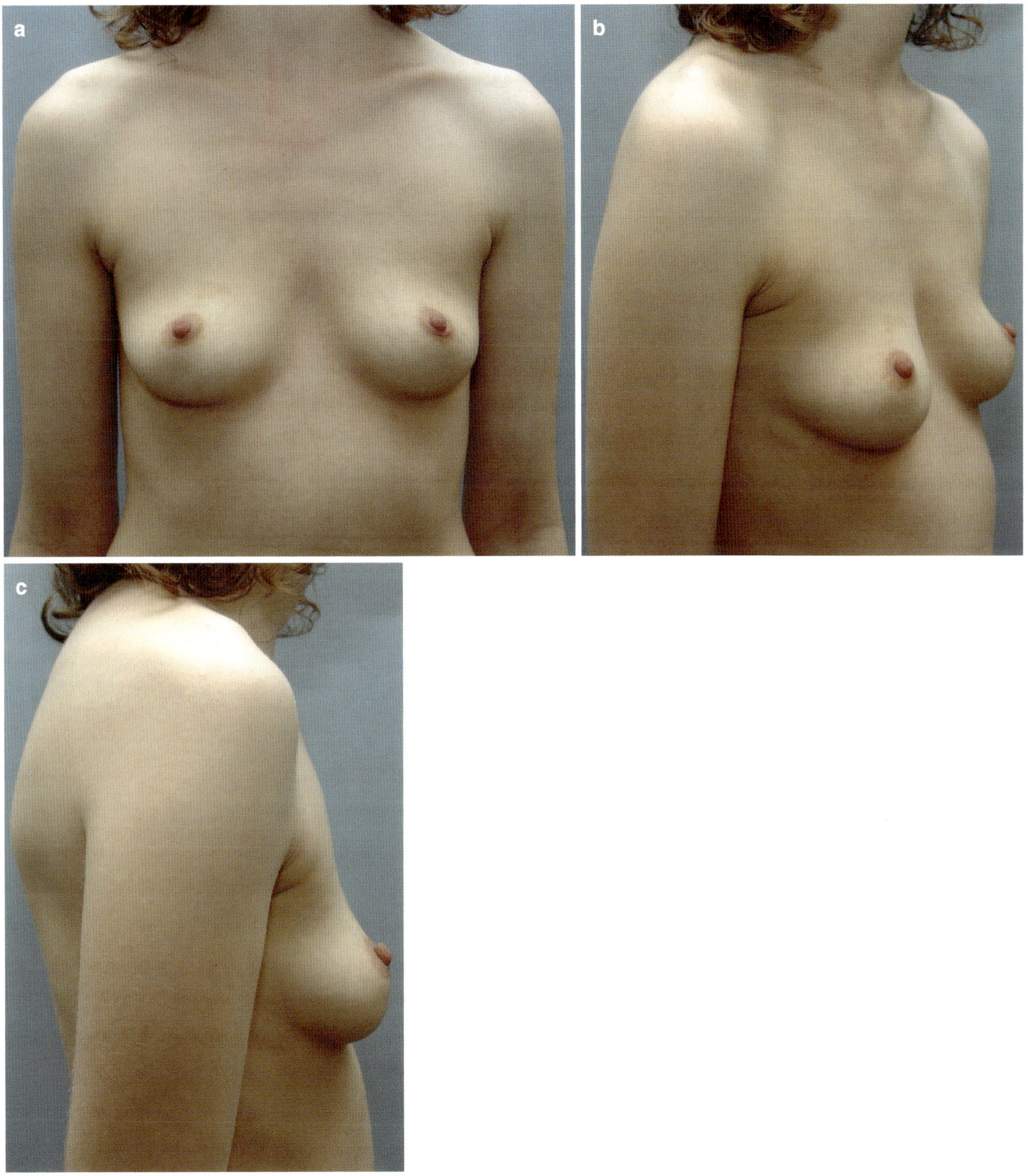

Fig. 5.14 (**a–c**) Preoperative photographs of a 36-year-old woman with A-cup bra size who desired breast augmentation surgery via a transaxillary endoscopic approach. Her goal was to become a C-cup

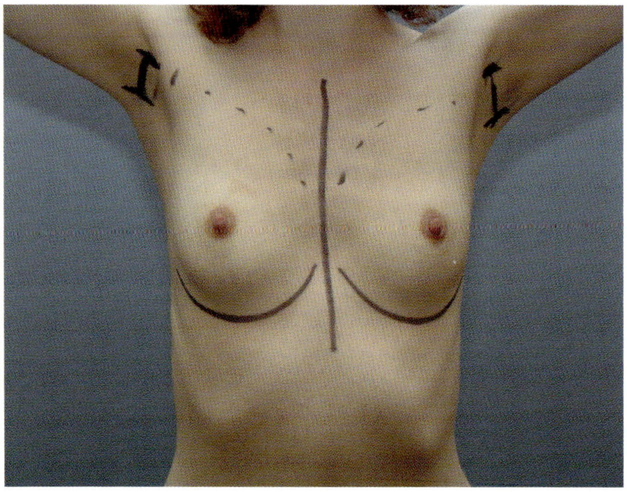

Fig. 5.15 Preoperative markings for the incisions and the areas of dissection are shown

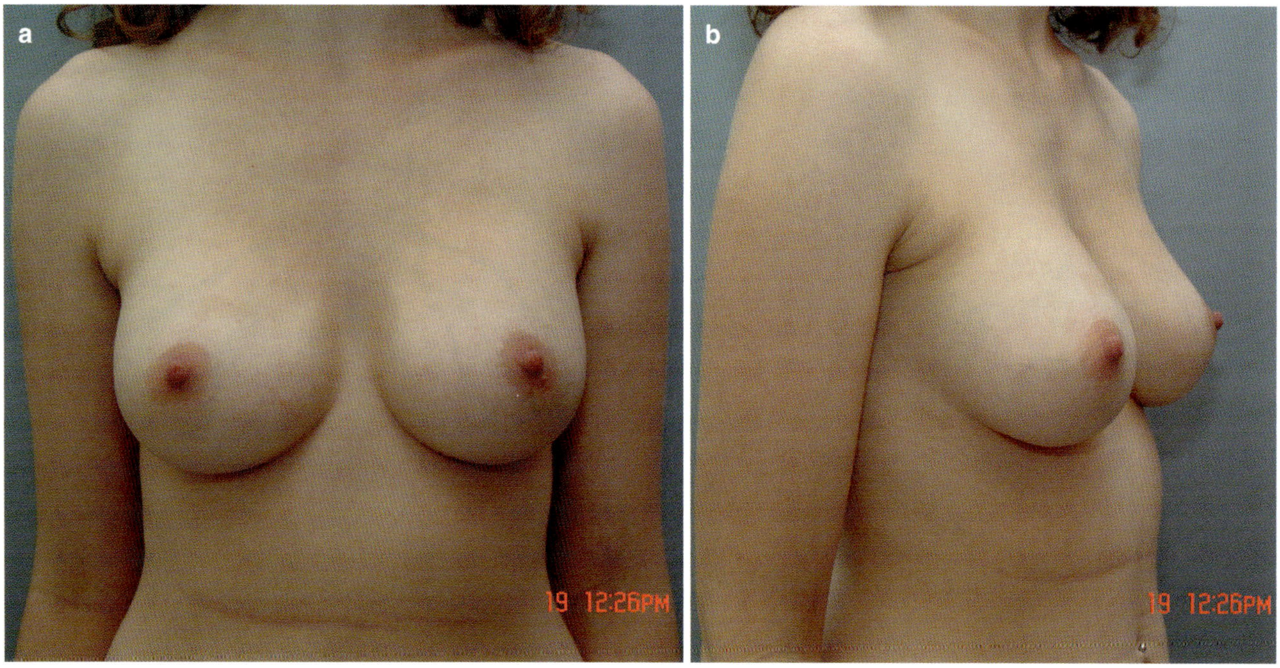

Fig. 5.16 (**a**–**e**) The same patient 14 months after transaxillary endoscopic subfascial breast augmentation with 286-mL Allergan Style 15 smooth silicone gel implants

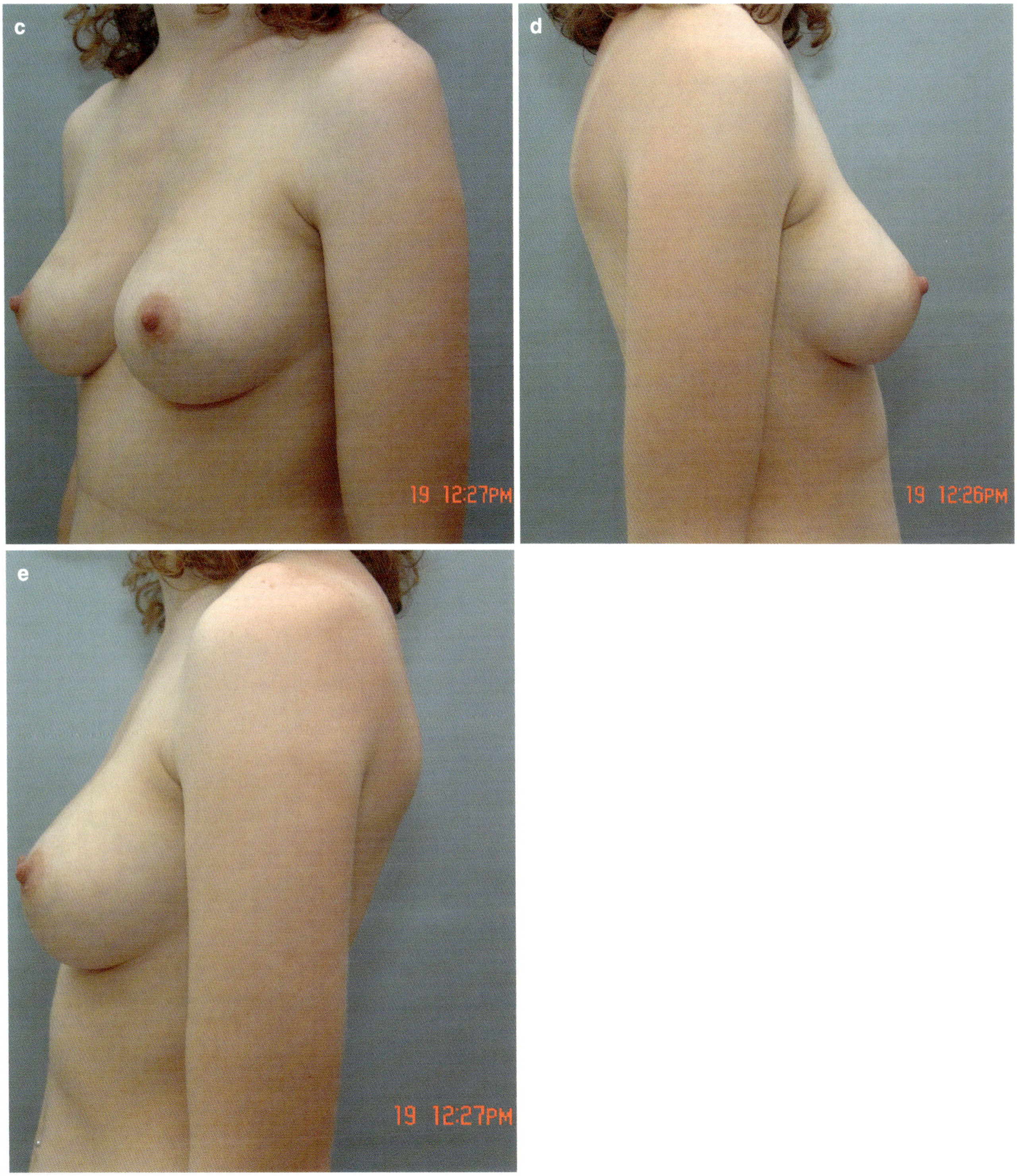

Fig. 5.16 (continued)

References

1. Price CI, Eaves FF, Nahai F, Jones G, Bostwick J. Endoscopic transaxillary subpectoral breast augmentation. Plast Reconstr Surg. 1994;94:612–9.
2. Strock LL. Transaxillary endoscopic silicone gel breast augmentation. Aesthet Surg J. 2010;30:745–55.
3. Graf RM, Bernardes A, Auersvald A, Darnasio RCC. Subfascial endoscopic transaxillary augmentation mammaplasty. Aesthetic Plast Surg. 2000;24:220–2.
4. Graf RM, Bernardes A, Rippel R, Araujo LR, Damasio RC, Auersvald A. Subfascial breast implant: a new procedure. Plast Reconstr Surg. 2003;111:904–8.
5. Serra-Renom JM, Garrido MF, Yoon T. Augmentation mammaplasty with anatomic soft, cohesive silicone implant using the transaxillary approach at a subfascial level with endoscopic assistance. Plast Reconstr Surg. 2005;116:640–5.
6. Hunstad JP, Webb LS. Subfascial breast augmentation: a comprehensive experience. Aesthetic Plast Surg. 2010;24:365–73.
7. Goes JC, Landecker A. Optimizing outcomes in breast augmentation: seven years of experience with the subfascial plane. Aesthetic Plast Surg. 2003;27:178–84.
8. Baxter RA. Subfascial breast augmentation: theme and variations. Aesthet Surg J. 2005;25:447–53.
9. Hwang K, Huan F, Hwang SW, Kim SH, Han SH. The course of the intercostobrachial nerve in the axillary region and as it is related to transaxillary breast augmentation. Ann Plast Surg. 2014;72:337–9.
10. Tebbetts JB. Axillary endoscopic breast augmentation: processes derived from a 28-year experience to optimize outcomes. Plast Reconstr Surg. 2006;118(Suppl):53S–80.
11. Giordano PA, Roif M, Laurent B, Mateu J. Endoscopic transaxillary breast augmentation: clinical evaluation of a series of 306 patients over a 9-year period. Aesthet Surg J. 2007;27:47–54.

Endoscope-Assisted Partial Mastectomy

6

Nobuyuki Takemoto, Ai Koyanagi, and Hiroshi Yamamoto

Breast-conserving therapy (BCT) is currently the mainstream treatment for stage I and stage II breast cancer. Two techniques are available for BCT: the conventional conservative method (CCM) and endoscopic surgery. Endoscopic surgery has the advantage of improving cosmetic outcome and early postoperative quality of life, and alleviating postoperative pain. Because cosmetic outcome can have a substantial psychological impact on women who undergo breast cancer surgery [1], it is imperative that methods to improve cosmetic outcome be developed, particularly for lower tumor location, as CCM performed in this location often leads to residual deformity [2–6]. Our endoscopic surgery, endoscope-assisted partial mastectomy (EAPM) with filling of the dead space using absorbable meshes (polyglactin and cellulose), is a new technique based on the method described by Yamagata and Iwai [7]. In contrast to CCM, which leaves a large surgical scar on the breast, EAPM can be performed via a small incision on the areola, leaving only an inconspicuous surgical scar. Thus, this method minimizes postoperative deformity.

We have previously reported that EAPM is superior to CCM for postoperative cosmetic outcomes, especially for lower tumor location [8]. In our study, satisfactory results were obtained for only 18.8 % of the patients who underwent CCM for lower tumor location, versus 68.6 % for upper location. The corresponding figures for EAPM were 57.9 % (lower location) and 78.1 % (upper location). EAPM was significantly superior to CCM for lower inner location (location B) (satisfactory results, 70.0 % vs. 12.5 %; $p=0.025$). As for individual analysis by each scoring factor (breast retraction assessment, nipple deviation, atrophy, skin change, scar), EAPM performed better than CCM in regards to atrophy and scar. This chapter introduces the surgical procedures of EAPM, together with a new dye method that we developed to identify sentinel lymph nodes (SLNs).

N. Takemoto, MD, PhD (✉)
Department of Breast and Endocrine Surgery, Japan Medical Alliance, Higashi Saitama General Hospital, 5-517 Yoshino, Satte, Saitama 340-0153, Japan
e-mail: monochrome-rainbow@iijmio-mail.jp

A. Koyanagi, MD, MSc, PhD
Research and Development Unit, Parc Sanitari Sant Joan de Déu, Fundació Sant Joan de Déu, Dr. Antoni Pujadas, 42 Sant Boi de Llobregat, Barcelona 08830, Spain
e-mail: a.koyanagi@pssjd.org

H. Yamamoto, MD, PhD
Geriatric Health Service Facility, Yokohama Brain and Spine Center, Japan Medical Alliance, 1-2-1, Takigashira, Isogoi-ku, Yokohama, Kanagawa 235-0012, Japan
e-mail: y_yamamoto@jin-ai.or.jp

E. Raposio (ed.), *Atlas of Endoscopic Plastic Surgery*, DOI 10.1007/978-3-319-19461-5_6

6.1 Surgical Technique

The patient is placed in a supine position on the operating table and a small pillow is placed under the back of the operating side of the patient. The arm on the surgical side is extended perpendicular to the body axis. The operator stands at the opposite side of the tumor, and the monitor is put at the tumor site. After the induction of general anesthesia and sterilization of the operation site, a combination of indocyanine green 10 mg (Daiichi-Sankyo; Tokyo, Japan) and 8 mg indigo carmine (Daiichi-Sankyo, Tokyo, Japan) is injected into the subareolar region for SLN biopsy (Fig. 6.1).

Next, the tumor is confirmed by means of 7.5-MHz ultrasonography, and a mixture of indigo carmine (12 mg) and xylocaine jelly 2 % (2–3 mL) (AstraZeneca; Tokyo, Japan) is injected to mark the resection line of the mammary gland at 12 point locations under ultrasound guidance, where the resection line is delineated further than 2.1 cm from the edge of the tumor. On the monitor, fluorescence images (Fig. 6.2) are obtained by using Photodynamic Eye (PDE) (Hamamatsu Photonics; Hamamatsu, SP, Japan), and subcutaneous lymphatic channels are usually detected over the skin within 1 or 2 min. When fluorescence images are poor, additional massage of the injection point is useful.

The subcutaneous lymphatic channels are marked on the skin, based on the PDE image (Fig. 6.3).

A 2-cm skin incision (Fig. 6.4) is made near the point of disappearance of the fluorescence under operating light conditions.

After skin incision, the subcutaneous fat tissues are dissected and the stained lymphatic channels are identified. Stained lymphatic channels are carefully dissected and traced until the first-drained lymph node is identified. The blue-stained SLNs are resected by direct visual inspection, together with the surrounding fatty tissue (Fig. 6.5). Usually, two or more lymph nodes are identified.

If blue-stained SLNs cannot be identified, the operating field is directly inspected using PDE, and the fluorescent lymph nodes are identified. Figure 6.6 illustrates a case in which the blue-stained lymph node could not be identified by direct visual inspection. Using the PDE, however, we were able to easily identify the SLN fluorescence on the monitor.

Fluorescence imaging is also used for postoperative SLN confirmation, and EAPM is performed while the resected SLNs are pathologically examined by hematoxylin and eosin (HE) stain with frozen section.

The periareolar incision is placed at about 120°. From the incision, a Visiport™ Plus Optical Trocar (Covidien; Mansfield, MA, USA) with a rigid endoscope (Fig. 6.7) is inserted to create a 160°-wide subcutaneous tunnel. The light at the tip of the Visiport™ is used to confirm that the tip is inserted parallel to the skin and the breast tissue is being detached (Fig. 6.8).

Using PowerStar Bipolar Scissors (Ethicon; Somerville, NJ, USA) or Harmonic scalpel (Ethicon Endo-Surgery; Cincinnati, OH, USA), the tissue between the tunnels is cut (Fig. 6.9), and a skin flap with a slight amount of fat is created.

A vertical incision is placed at the marking point closest to the nipple, using an electrocautery to expose and cut the pectoralis major fascia. Between the fascia and the muscle, a Round-Preperitoneal Distention Balloon (PDB) (Covidien; Mansfield, MA, USA) is inserted, and the mammary gland is separated from the pectoralis major muscle (Fig. 6.10). The balloon is inflated for 5 min (Fig. 6.11) and also serves for hemostasis.

At this stage, the direct-vision scope is inserted into the balloon. If the PDB is inserted properly, the muscle fibers of the pectoralis major muscle can be identified on the monitor.

The next step is excision of the tumor. The nipple is covered with gauzes to prevent it from being burnt, and the location of the tumor is reconfirmed by palpation. Using an electrocautery, the mammary gland is cut vertically while connecting the marking points, so that the excised tumor is a cylindrical mass (Fig. 6.12).

After thorough hemostasis, the mastectomized area is slightly sutured without inducing breast deformation. Vicryl® mesh (15 × 15 cm, Ethicon; Somerville, NJ, USA) wrapped in Gynecare Interceed™ (7.6 × 10.2 cm; Ethicon) is used to fill the remaining dead space (Fig. 6.13).

The number of meshes depends on the resection volume. We fill the mesh loosely until the breast on the operative side is not dented in the supine position and symmetry of both breasts is achieved (Fig. 6.14).

The surgical wound is closed by placing subcutaneous buried sutures using 5-0 PDS-II clear (Ethicon Endo-Surgery; Cincinnati, OH, USA).

The cosmetic outcome of patients who underwent EAPM is shown in Fig. 6.15a, b. Near symmetry of the breasts can be seen in both cases.

In general, EAPM can be performed in all cases where BCT is indicated. The exceptions are cases with tumors fixed to the skin or muscle, as EAPM applies skin-sparing partial mastectomy. Location of the tumor more than 10 cm away from the nipple is considered a relative contraindication because tissue detachment becomes too extensive with the periareolar approach, and sufficient detachment may not be achieved. The important advantage associated with the periareolar approach—the lack of a skin incision on the breast—thus may be undermined. In addition, although EAPM improves cosmetic outcome in BCT for tumors of lower location in general, its performance may be limited in cases where the tumor is located in the lower-outer quadrant (location D). We have been unable to make firm conclusions regarding the utility of EAPM for tumors in this location [8], and we think that further investigation is necessary.

Among other benefits, EAPM has the advantage of not requiring reconstruction, as in oncoplastic surgery [9–11]. To fill the dead space after tumor resection, we use two types of absorbable meshes: Vicryl® mesh and Interceed™. The former, composed of poly-L-lactic acid, requires 6 months to 1 year to dissolve and be absorbed [12]. The latter, a well-known material used in abdominal surgery, is composed of oxidized regenerated cellulose; it dissolves and is absorbed in 1–2 months [12]. The dead space becomes filled with the absorbable meshes plus reactive tissue fluid within 2–3 days after the insertion of the Vicryl® mesh wrapped in Interceed™. Foreign-body reaction occurs and promotes granulation and the formation of connective tissue along the margin of the dead space. Within 1–2 months after the surgery, the margin becomes suitably hard and the dead space forms a comparatively fixed shape [12, 13]. Interceed™ prevents the adhesion of the Vicryl® mesh to the wall of the dead space and retraction of the skin into the dead space.

Complications associated with the mesh can occur, such as infection or overproduction of fluid induced by the absorbable meshes. We previously reported the rate of mesh infection to be 11.2 %; all those who had mesh infection had unsatisfactory cosmetic outcomes and had their mesh removed [8]. To reduce the infection rates, we introduced four new measures: (1) preoperative and postoperative antibiotics drip; (2) glove exchange before mesh insertion; (3) thorough washing of the dead space before mesh insertion; and (4) avoidance of EAPM in patients with uncontrolled diabetes mellitus, autoimmune disease, or steroid use. These measures halved the incidence of mesh infection but did not eliminate it entirely.

In our institution, SLN biopsy is performed with the mixed dye method using PDE. This method is basically the same as the dye method, but the PDE is used in conjunction with the dye for preoperative identification of lymphatic channels, incision location, and intraoperative detection of nonstained SLNs [14]. This method is simple, reliable, and cost-effective, and is also feasible in institutions where the use of radioisotopes is limited.

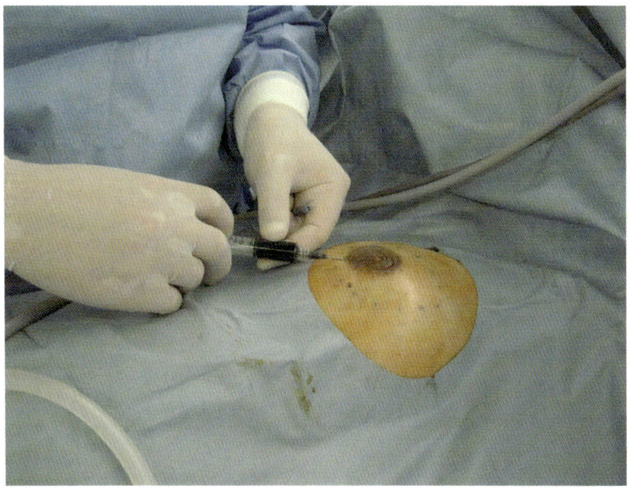

Fig. 6.1 Dye injection into the subareolar region for sentinel lymph node biopsy

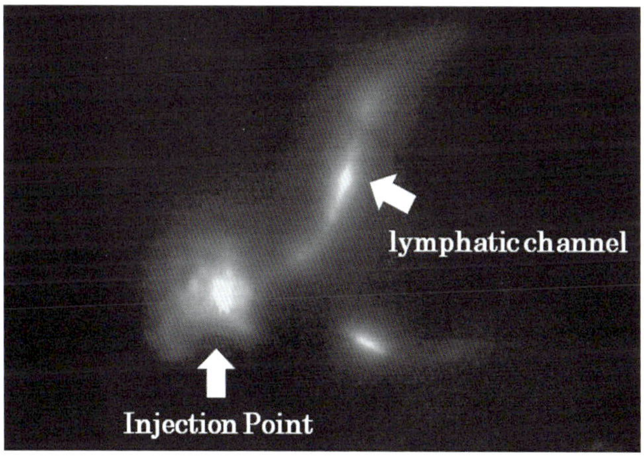

Fig. 6.2 Fluorescence images of the lymphatic channel on the monitor

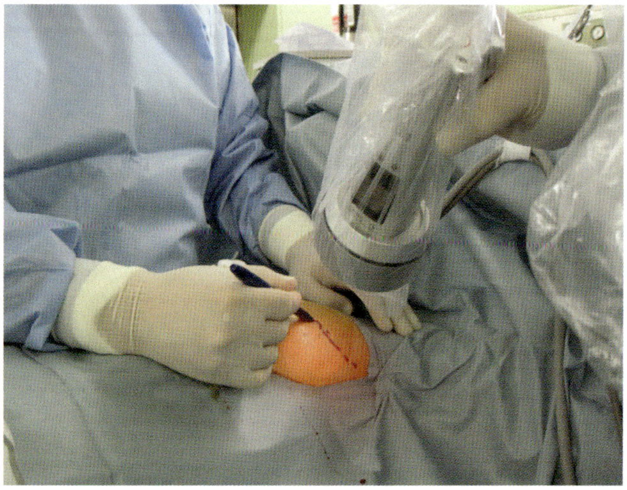

Fig. 6.3 Lymphatic channel marking on the skin based on Photodynamic Eye images

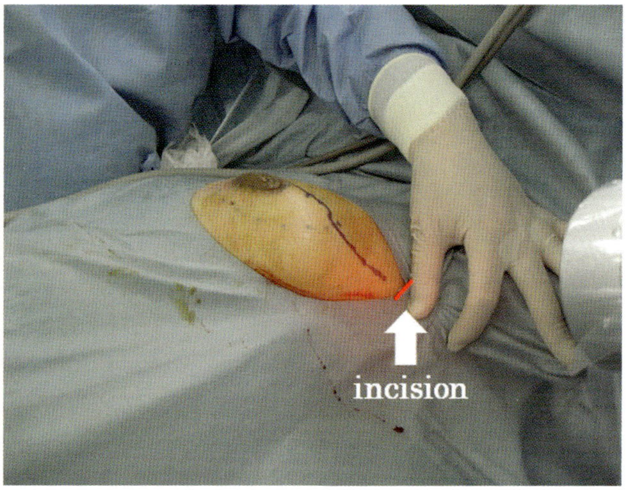

Fig. 6.4 Skin incision for sentinel lymph node biopsy

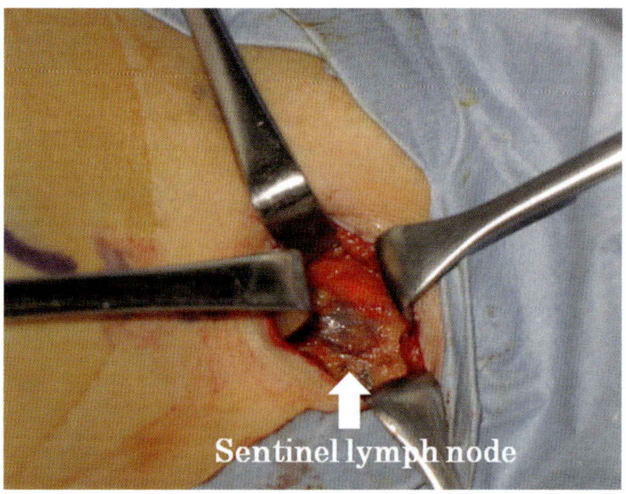

Fig. 6.5 Blue-stained sentinel lymph node

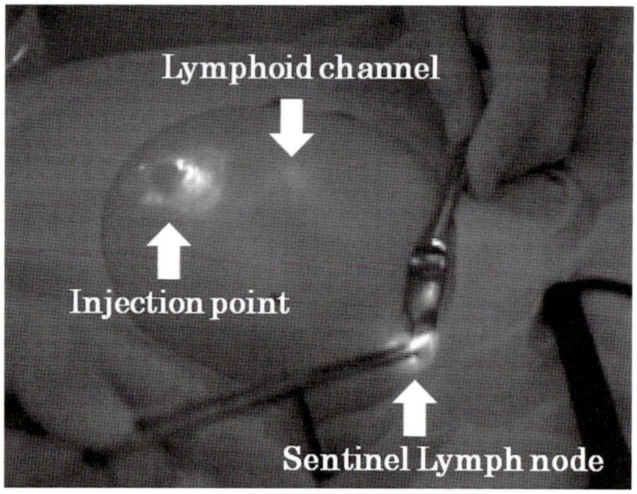

Fig. 6.6 Fluorescence image of operative field

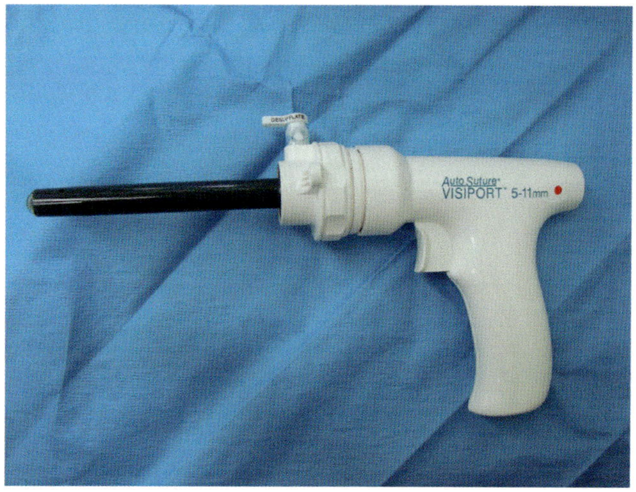

Fig. 6.7 Visiport™ optical trocar

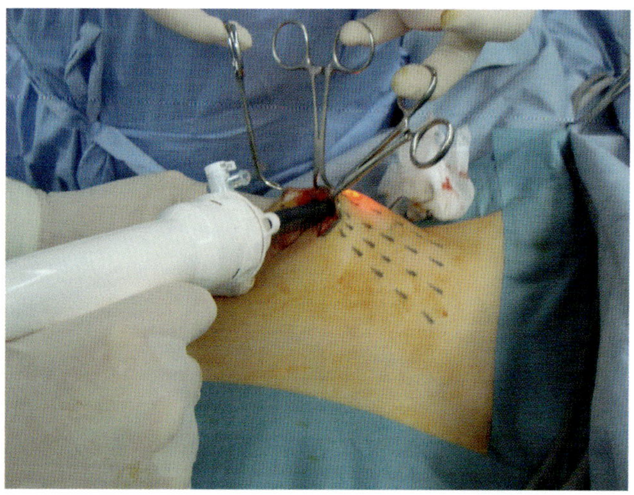

Fig. 6.8 Detachment of subcutaneous tissue using Visiport™

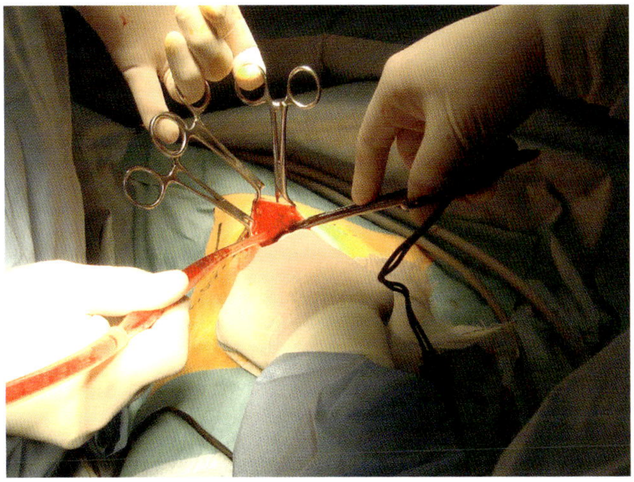

Fig. 6.9 Subcutaneous tunnel cutting using PowerStar Bipolar Scissors or Harmonic scalpel

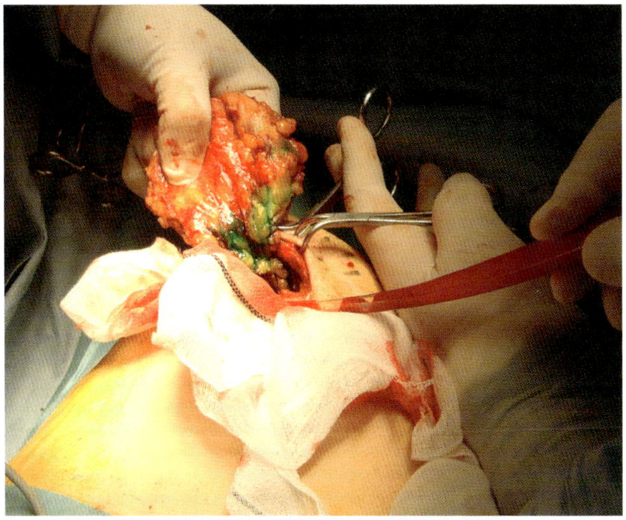

Fig. 6.12 Partial resection of mammary gland using an electrocautery

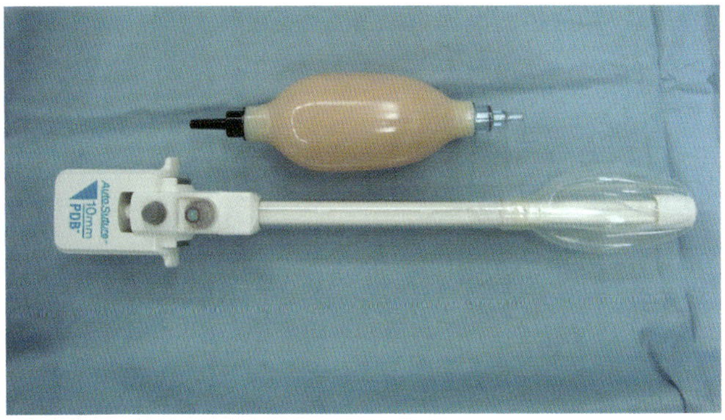

Fig. 6.10 Round-Preperitoneal Distention Balloon

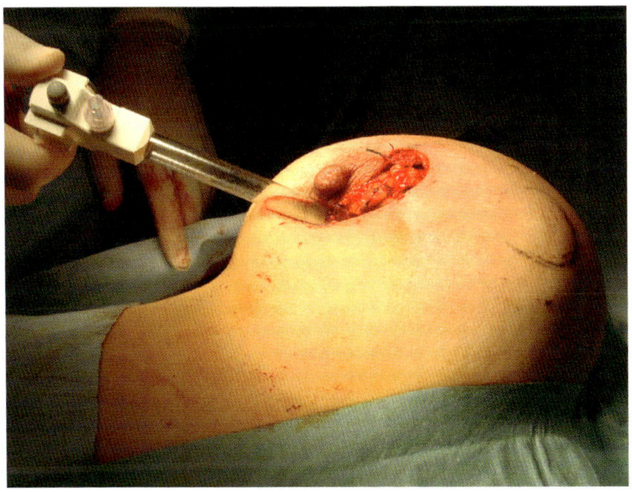

Fig. 6.11 Inflation of the Preperitoneal Distention Balloon

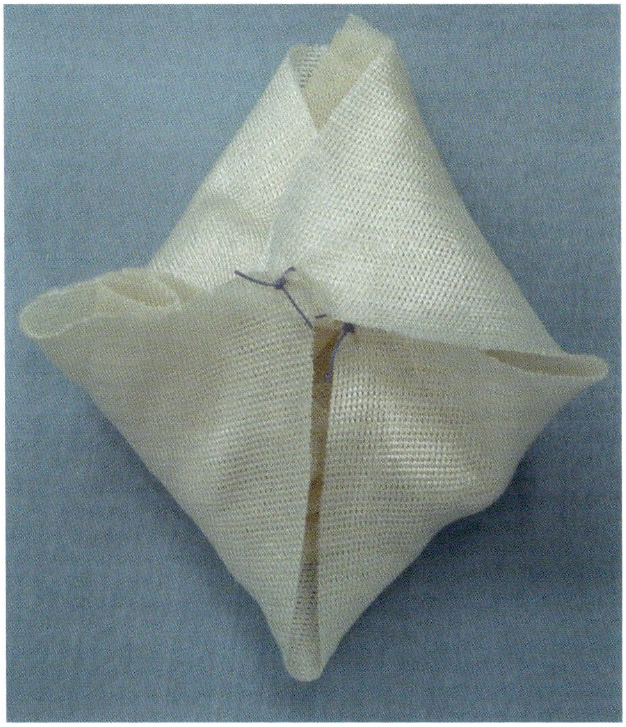

Fig. 6.13 Inserted mesh (Vicryl® mesh wrapped in Interceed™)

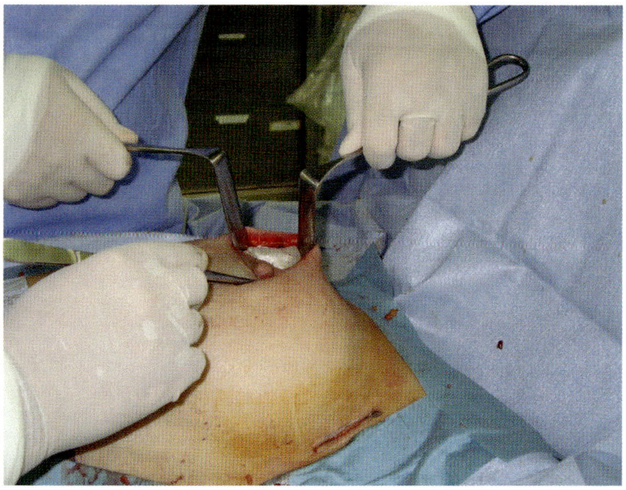

Fig. 6.14 Mesh insertion in the mastectomized area

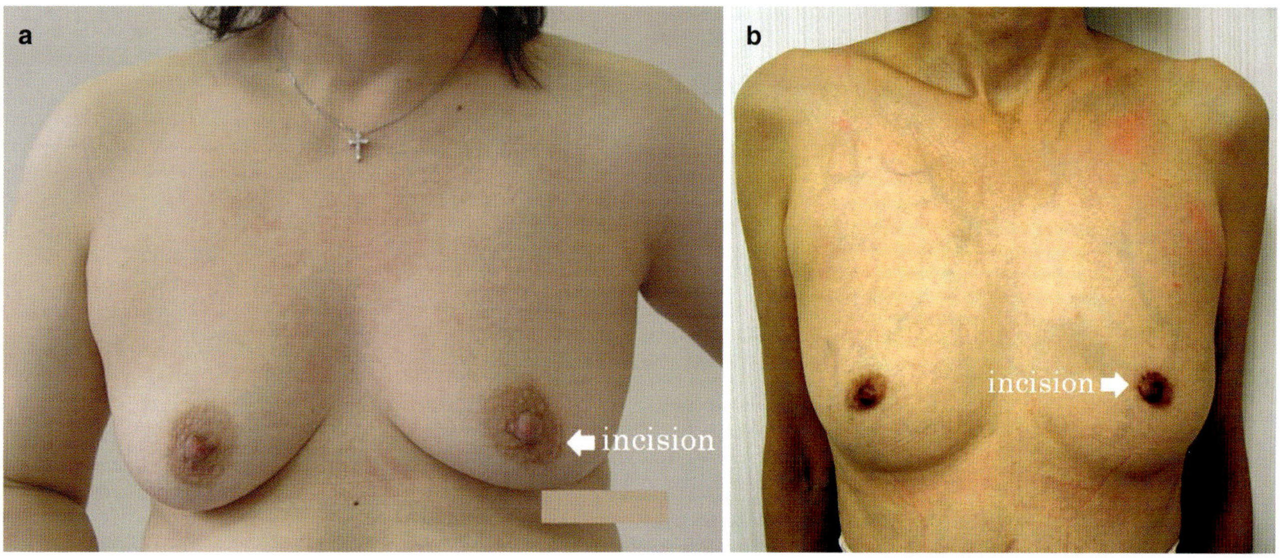

Fig. 6.15 The cosmetic outcome of patients who underwent endoscope-assisted partial mastectomy (EAPM). (**a**), A 47-year-old woman shown 3 years after surgery. The tumor (invasive ductal carcinoma, size 22 × 25 × 12 mm) was located at the 3 o'clock position in the left breast. (**b**), A 55-year-old woman 5 years after surgery. The tumor (invasive ductal carcinoma, size 18 × 25 × 22 mm) was located at the 11 o'clock position in the left breast

Conclusions

The unique feature of EAPM is the maintenance of cosmetic outcome by insertion of absorbable meshes without unnecessary skin incisions or excisions, as in radical BCT. EAPM has the advantage of not requiring reconstruction, as in oncoplastic surgery, and has the additional benefits of simplicity and cost-effectiveness.

Although CCM often leads to residual deformity for lower tumor locations, EAPM can improve cosmetic outcome, especially for tumors in location B. The performance of EAPM for tumors in location D is limited, however, and we believe that other procedures should also be considered for tumors in this location.

The major complication of EAPM is mesh infection. As mesh infection leads to unsatisfactory cosmetic outcomes, its prevention is of vital importance. Although preventive measures have decreased the infection rate, it has not yet been reduced to null. Further investigation of measures to prevent mesh infection is necessary.

References

1. Al-Ghazal SK, Fallowfield L, Blamey RW. Does cosmetic outcome from treatment of primary breast cancer influence psychosocial morbidity? Eur J Surg Oncol. 1999;25:571–3.
2. Clough KB, Nos C, Salmon RJ, Soussaline M, Durand JC. Conservative treatment of breast cancers by mammaplasty and irradiation: a new approach to lower quadrant tumors. Plast Reconstr Surg. 1995;96:363–70.
3. Rose MA, Olivotto I, Cady B, Koufman C, Osteen R, Silver B, et al. Conservative surgery and radiation therapy for early breast cancer. Long-term cosmetic results. Arch Surg. 1989;124:153–7.
4. Liljegren G, Holmberg L, Westman G. The cosmetic outcome in early breast cancer treated with sector resection with or without radiotherapy. Uppsala-Orebro Breast Cancer Study Group. Eur J Cancer. 1993;29A:2083–9.
5. Sarin R, Dinshaw KA, Shrivastava SK, Sharma V, Deore SM. Therapeutic factors influencing the cosmetic outcome and late complications in the conservative management of early breast cancer. Int J Radiat Oncol Biol Phys. 1993;27:285–92.
6. Van Limbergen E, Rijnders A, van der Schueren E, Lerut T, Christiaens R. Cosmetic evaluation of breast conserving treatment for mammary cancer. 2. A quantitative analysis of the influence of radiation dose, fractionation schedules and surgical treatment techniques on cosmetic results. Radiother Oncol. 1989;16:253–67.
7. Yamagata M, Iwai S. Endoscopic treatment for breast cancer [in Japanese]. J Jpn Soc Endosc Surg. 1997;2:272–7.
8. Takemoto N, Koyanagi A, Yamamoto H. Comparison between endoscope-assisted partial mastectomy with filling of dead space using absorbable mesh and conventional conservative method on cosmetic outcome in patients with stage I or II breast cancer. Surg Laparosc Endosc Percutan Tech. 2012;22:68–72.
9. Hernanz F, Regaño S, Redondo-Figuero C, Orallo V, Erasun F, Gómez-Fleitas M. Oncoplastic breast-conserving surgery: analysis of quadrantectomy and immediate reconstruction with latissimus dorsi flap. World J Surg. 2007;31:1934–40.
10. Thomson HJ, Potter S, Greenwood RJ, Bahl A, Barker J, Cawthorn SJ, Winters ZE. A prospective longitudinal study of cosmetic outcome in immediate latissimus dorsi breast reconstruction and the influence of radiotherapy. Ann Surg Oncol. 2008;15:1081–91.
11. Ho WS, Ying SY, Chan AC. Endoscopic-assisted subcutaneous mastectomy and axillary dissection with immediate mammary prosthesis reconstruction for early breast cancer. Surg Endosc. 2002;16:302–6.
12. Sanuki J, Fukuma E. Volume replacement for correcting breast deformity after breast conserving surgery [in Japanese]. Surgery. 2007;69:2007–10.
13. Sanuki J, Fukuma E, Wadamori K, Higa K, Sakamoto N, Tsunoda Y. Volume replacement with polyglycolic acid mesh for correcting breast deformity after endoscopic conservative surgery. Clin Breast Cancer. 2005;6:175.
14. Takemoto N, Koyanagi A, Yamamoto H, Shimura K, Fujii R. Comparison of the indocyanine green dye method versus the combined method of indigo carmine blue dye with indocyanine green fluorescence imaging for sentinel lymph node biopsy in patients with stage I or II breast cancer. Ann Oncol. 2014;25 Suppl 1:i3.

7 Breast Reconstruction Using Laparoscopically Harvested Omental Flap

Hisamitsu Zaha

Recently, the omentum has attracted much attention for its immunological and angiogenic features. Many applications for the omentum have been reported because of its protective role against infection and regenerative properties that are beneficial for ischemia. Kiricuta [1] was the first to use pedicled omental flaps in a range of indications including breast cancer surgery. Surprisingly, various new indications such as chronic spinal cord injury and Alzheimer's disease have also emerged [2]. Nevertheless, the use of the omental flap has not obtained widespread popularity because of the need for laparotomy, but rapid advances in endoscopic surgery now allow laparoscopic harvesting of the omental flap with less donor-site deformity and morbidity [3], thus making the use of the omental flap more attractive.

Breast-conserving surgery (BCS) is still a standard surgical modality as a treatment of choice in early breast cancer. With wider excision, however, the risk of breast deformity, disfigurement, and patient dissatisfaction increases. A volume replacement technique is often needed for smaller breasts or for patients with a small breast-to-tumor ratio. The latissimus dorsi (LD) flap plays a main role in volume replacement, but has the disadvantages of donor-site morbidity and deformity, such as seroma formation [4]. Perforator flaps, including the thoracodorsal artery perforator (TDAP) flap and the intercostal artery perforator (ICAP) flap have been developed to minimize these problems [5], but the locations to which they are adaptable are limited.

Laparoscopic harvest of the omental flap compensates for the donor-site disadvantages of other flaps [6–8] and can preserve the LD and/or the deep inferior epigastric perforator (DIEP) flaps for future total reconstruction.

7.1 Indications

- Breast reconstruction immediately after BCS or nipple-sparing mastectomy (NSM) in patients with stage 0, I, or II breast cancer.
  - For BCS, the omental flap is used when a 20 % or wider region of the breast tissue is resected or the cosmetic result is poor because of the location of the tumor in the medial quadrants.
  - For NSM, the procedure is applicable only to selected patients because the volume of the omental flap may be inadequate for total reconstruction. The use of an implant covered with the omental flap is one good option for immediate reconstruction after NSM.
- Delayed repair of a partial mastectomy deformity.
- Partial reconstruction for benign breast disorders such as giant fibroadenoma or phylloides tumor.

7.2 Contraindications

- History of intra-abdominal malignancy or upper abdominal laparotomy. Patients with a history of laparoscopic surgery (e.g., laparoscopic cholecystectomy) or lower abdominal surgery (e.g., Caesarean section) should not be excluded.
- Body mass index (BMI) of 35 kg/m^2 or more.

H. Zaha, MD
Department of Breast Surgery, Nakagami Hospital,
6-25-5 Chibana, Okinawa-City, Okinawa 904-2195, Japan
e-mail: hisamitu@nakagami.or.jp

E. Raposio (ed.), *Atlas of Endoscopic Plastic Surgery*, DOI 10.1007/978-3-319-19461-5_7

7.3 Surgical Technique

7.3.1 Laparoscopic Harvesting of the Omental Flap

Surgery is performed with the patient under general anesthesia in the supine position, with the bilateral limbs abducted at 90°. A camera port (5 or 10 mm, 30°) is inserted through a transumbilicus incision with the surgeon positioned at the right side of the patient. Pneumoperitoneum is maintained at 8–10 mmHg. Two 5-mm ports for the surgical instruments are inserted from the right abdominal wall, one through the right upper quadrant at the level of a wedge of the rectus muscle, and the other through the right lateral lower quadrant. One 5-mm port for the assistant is inserted through the left lateral lower quadrant (Fig. 7.1a).

First, the omentum is evaluated for size and adhesion (Fig. 7.1b) and is moved cephalic for dissection from the transverse colon.

The patient is placed in reverse Trendelenburg position with a right lateral oblique rotation. Usually a site slightly left of the center of the transverse colon is the most suitable place for starting dissection, providing easier access to the omental bursa (Fig. 7.2a).

To ensure that the omental bursa is entered successfully, a posterior wall of the stomach must be identified (Fig. 7.2b).

This step is very important for safe and successful harvesting of the omental flap. Then the dissection is advanced leftward while maintaining appropriate tension between the omentum and the transverse colon. Care is taken not to injure the transverse colon, especially near the splenic flexure (Fig. 7.2c).

After the splenocolic ligament is divided, the resection turns to the lower pole of the spleen, with great care not to tear the splenic capsule (Fig. 7.3a).

During the resection of the gastrosplenic ligament, the left gastroepiploic artery and vein (GEAV) are encountered. They can be resected with a laparoscopic coagulating shears (LCS) without ligation or clipping (Fig. 7.3b).

Because the right gastroepiploic artery is predominant, we always select the right gastroepiploic artery and vein as a pedicle. The more volume of the flap is needed, the more resection of the gastrosplenic ligament beyond the short gastric vessels must be performed. However, the left side of the omentum beyond the resection wedge of the left gastroepiploic artery tends to lack adequate vascular supply.

After complete division of the left side of the omentum, the gastric branches of the GEAV are divided, little by little, at a site as close to the stomach wall as possible, towards the pyloric ring (Fig. 7.4a).

Attention is paid to the main trunks of the GEAV, because they sometimes run very close to the stomach wall, and they can be difficult to identify when abundant fat deposit of the omentum is evident. Therefore, the gastric branches of the GEAV are pulled and stretched so that they run at a right angle to the stomach wall (Fig. 7.4b).

The dissection from the right side of the transverse colon is then advanced (Fig. 7.5a), and fusion between the posterior leaf of the gastrocolic ligament and the anterior leaf of the transverse mesocolon is carefully divided toward the anterior capsule of the pancreas head (Fig. 7.5b).

Upward traction of the omentum is maintained, and careful sharp and blunt dissection between the gastrocolic ligament and the transverse mesocolon is advanced until the roots of the GEAV are confirmed. Adhesion to the anterior wall of the duodenum is also carefully dissected and advanced to the root of the GEAV.

After complete dissection from the transverse colon, dissection from the stomach is advanced across the pyloric ring (Fig. 7.6a).

Very careful dissection is required at this point, because the GEAV run close to the wall of the stomach and the proximal duodenum, and the branches tend to bleed easily. It is better to resect as much fat tissue around the root of the GEAV as possible for the thin pedicle of the flap, to avoid the subsequent complication of ventral hernia. One of the epiploic vessels that descends on the right side of the omentum sometimes must be resected to make the longer pedicle. Then a pedicled omental flap is completed (Fig. 7.6b).

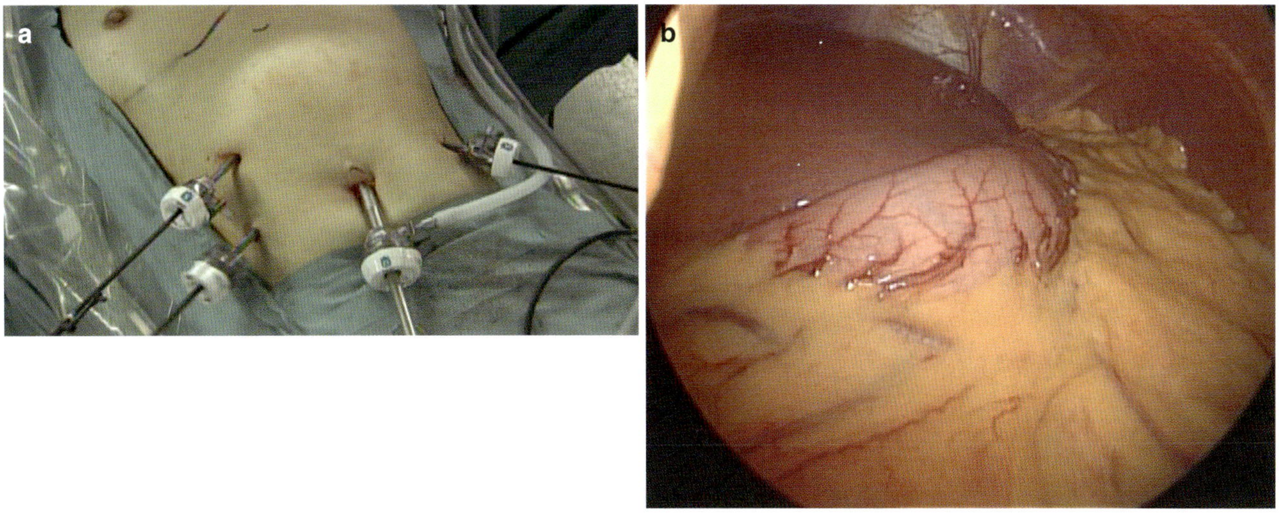

Fig. 7.1 (**a**) A camera port and two to three 5-mm ports are inserted. Care must be taken not to injure the epigastric vessels, not only to avoid hemorrhagic complications but also to allow the potential for future total reconstruction. (**b**) The omentum is evaluated for size and adhesion. Then the patient is placed in reverse Trendelenburg position with a right lateral oblique rotation

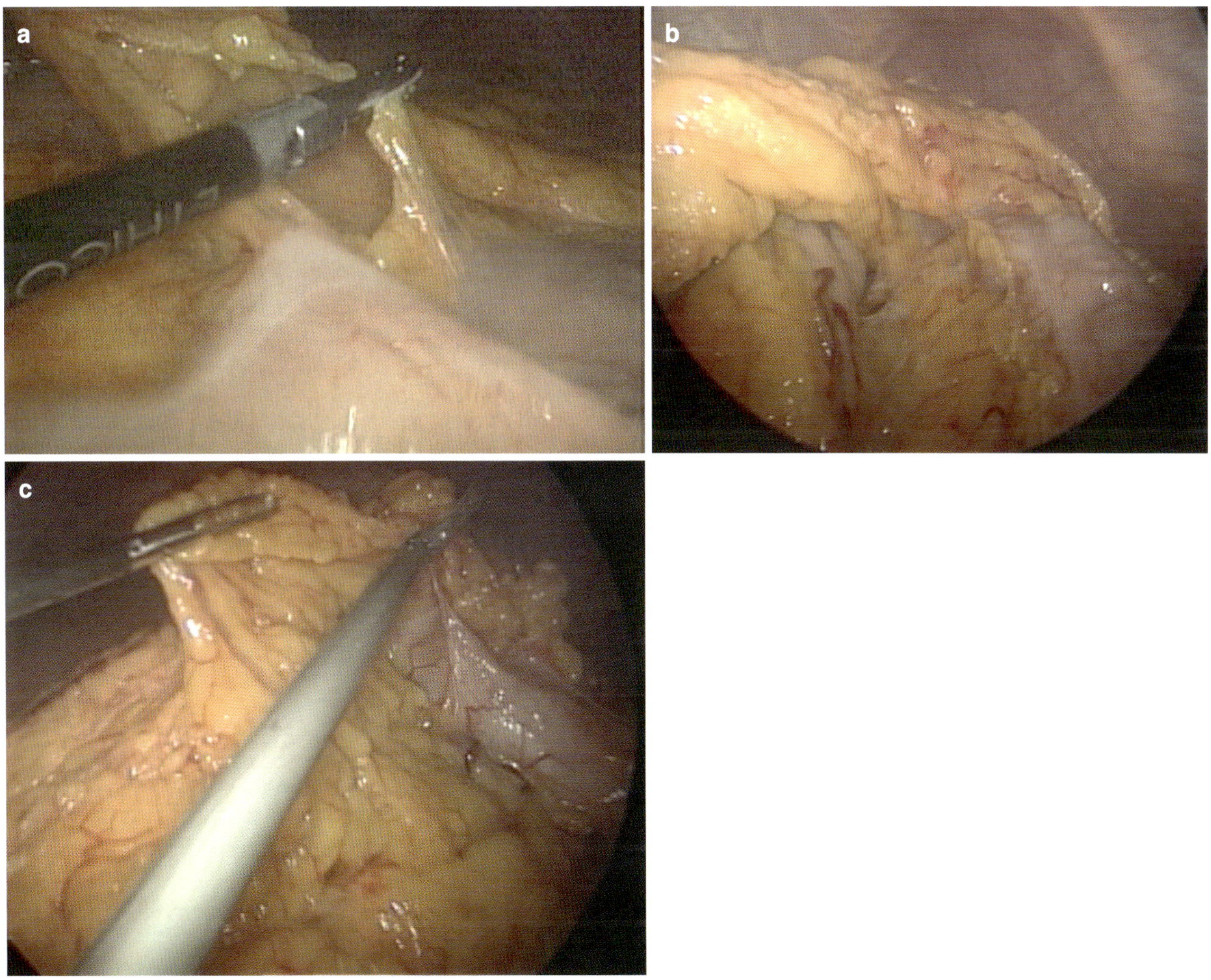

Fig. 7.2 (**a**) A site slightly left of the center of the transverse colon is the most suitable place for entering into the omental bursa. (**b**) To prevent injury of the omental flap, the posterior wall of the stomach must be identified in the first step of dissection. (**c**) Great care must be taken not to injure the transverse colon, not only by mechanical injury from grasping but also by thermal injury caused by the laparoscopic coagulating shears (LCS), especially near the splenic flexure

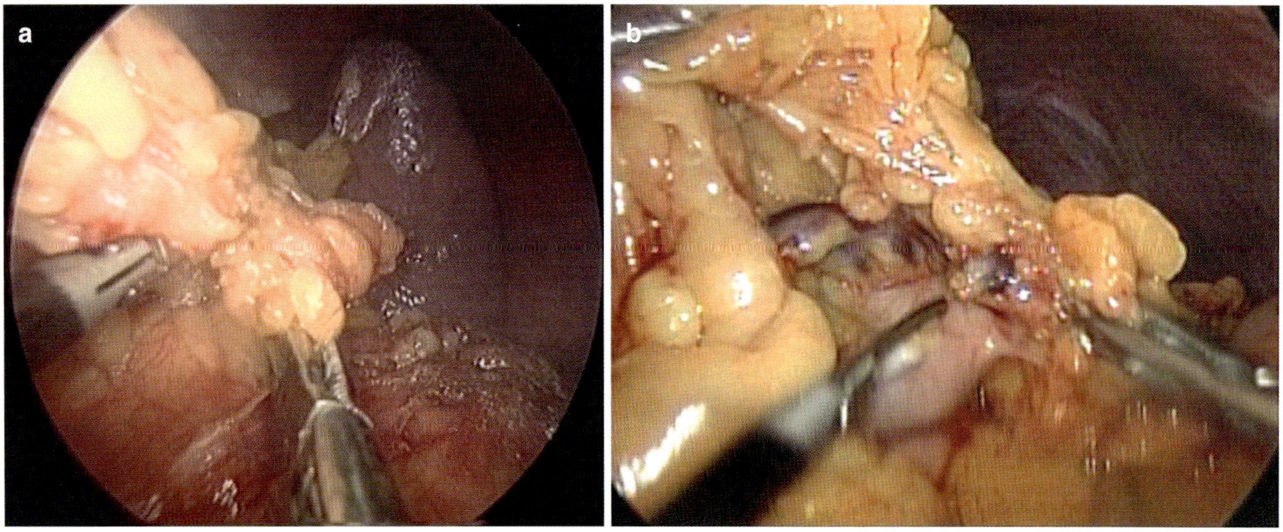

Fig. 7.3 (**a**) Transection of the left side of the omentum. After the splenocolic ligament is divided, the resection turns to the lower pole of the spleen, taking great care not to tear the splenic capsule. (**b**) The left gastroepiploic vessels can be resected with the LCS without ligation or clipping

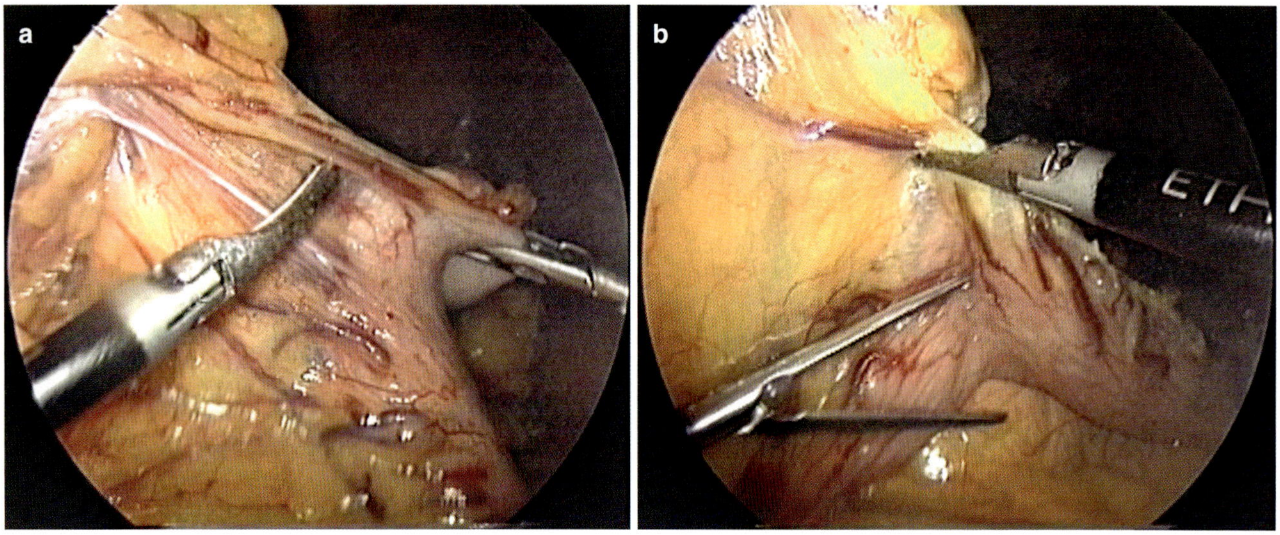

Fig. 7.4 (**a**) Unlike the transverse colon, the wall of the stomach is thick and strong. Then, the gastric branches of the gastroepiploic vessels should be divided at a site as close to the stomach wall as possible. (**b**) The gastric branches are pulled and stretched so as not to injure the main trunks of the gastroepiploic vessels

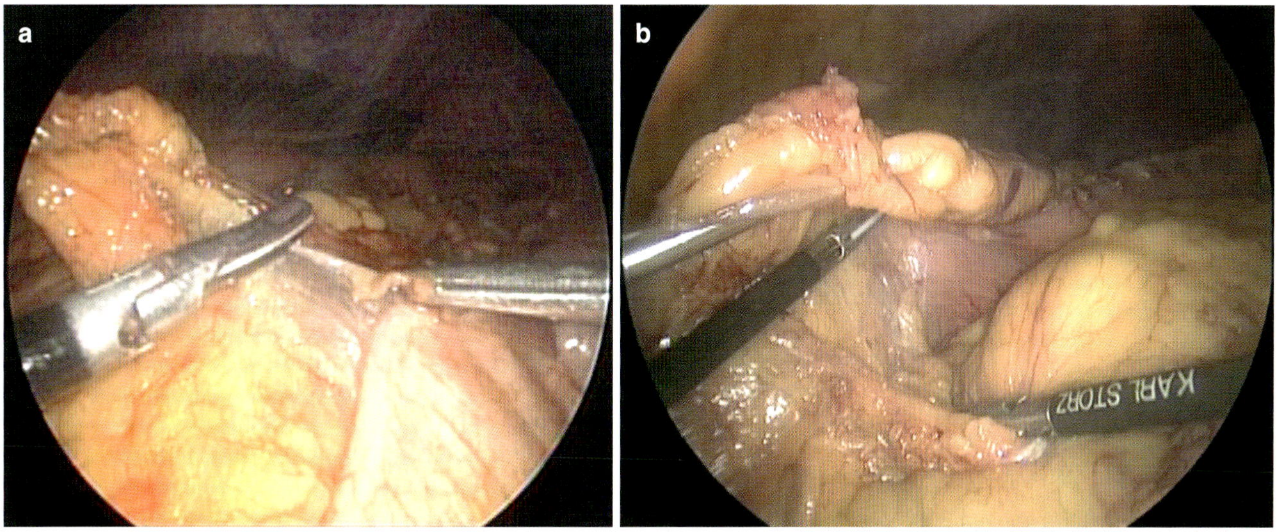

Fig. 7.5 (**a**) The dissection from the right side of the transverse colon is advanced with a left lateral oblique rotation. (**b**) Fusion between the posterior leaf of the gastrocolic ligament and the anterior leaf of the transverse mesocolon is bluntly divided with upward retraction of the stomach and downward retraction of the transverse mesocolon

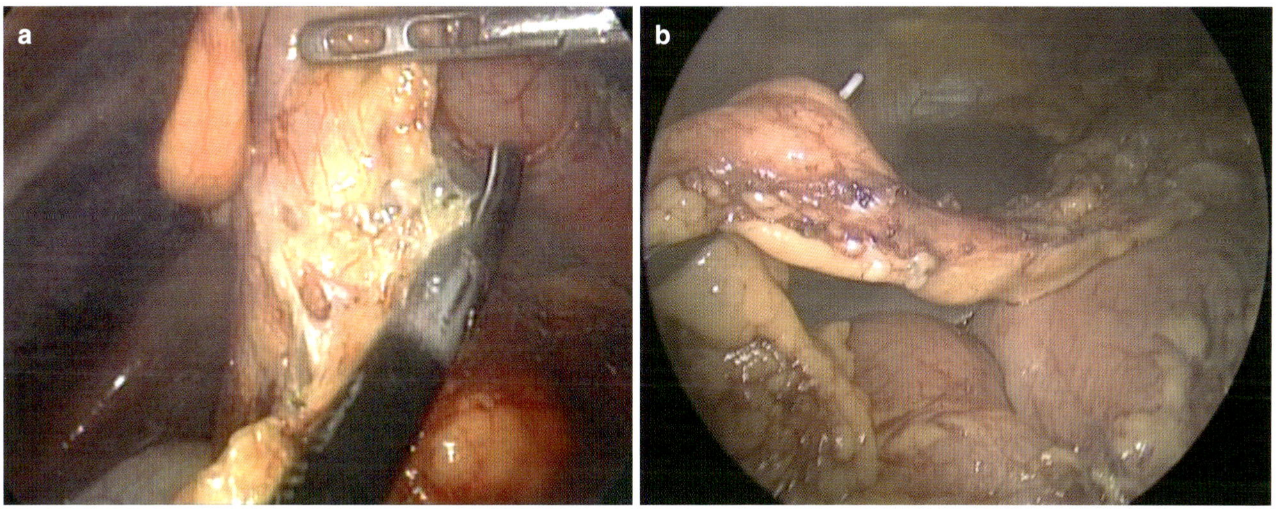

Fig. 7.6 (**a**) Resection of the gastric branches of the gastroepiploic vessels around the pyloric ring. (**b**) The root of the gastroepiploic vessels

7.3.2 Partial Breast Reconstruction After BCS

Using various skin incisions, the omental flap can be applied to any quadrants of partial mastectomy defects. For the lower quadrants, an inframammary skin incision is preferable (Fig. 7.7a, b).

After partial mastectomy, a subcutaneous tunnel about two fingerbreadths in width is prepared from an incision along the inframammary fold toward the xiphoidal process (Fig. 7.8a). When it reaches the white line, a longitudinal incision measuring 2 or 2.5 fingerbreadths is made to communicate with the abdominal cavity.

This communication is facilitated by intra-abdominal resection of the white line with the LCS (Fig. 7.8b, c).

For reconstruction of the right breast, the right side of the falciform ligament is resected to communicate with the tunnel, and vice versa for the left breast. The forceps or fingers are inserted into the abdominal cavity, and the pedicled omental flap is carefully withdrawn, avoiding twisting (Fig. 7.9a–d).

The omental flap can reach any quadrants of the breasts. Especially, volume replacements for the medial quadrants, which are difficult with the use of other autologous flaps, are comfortable fields for the omental flap (Fig. 7.10).

When the omental flap is large, a wider longitudinal abdominal incision and/or a small, transverse resection of the rectus muscles is added. When the incision is wider than two fingers, semiclosure of the abdominal incision is necessary after the flap is pulled out, to avoid incisional hernia. Hemostasis is carefully confirmed, and if the flap is too large to fill the defect of the breast, the excess amount of the omentum is resected. Subcutaneous fat around the tunnel and fat tissue around the pedicle are resected to avoid subcutaneous bulging due to the pedicle.

The cephalic and lateral cut margin of residual breast tissue is fixed with the pectoralis major muscle to avoid movement of the omental flap. It is important that the width of the pedicle and the entrance of the subcutaneous tunnel are small (<2 cm), to allow proper re-creation of the inframammary fold and avoid subcutaneous bulging (Fig. 7.11a).

Finally, the omental flap is placed over the pectoralis major muscle to fill the dead space in the breast tissue (Fig. 7.11b).

Fixation of the omental flap to the chest wall is usually unnecessary. A closed suction drain is inserted over the omental flap and the wound is closed in layers. Figure 7.11c–e illustrate the resulting minimal scarring and natural appearance.

The clinical cases in which partial mastectomy was performed in the lower quadrants shown in Figs. 7.12 and 7.13 show similarly excellent results.

For the upper quadrants, a periareolar incision is our preference. After partial mastectomy, an additional small incision is made on the medial inframammary fold to extract the omental flap (Fig. 7.14a–c).

A subglandular tunnel passing under the lower inner quadrant is also created between the inframammary incision and the partial mastectomy defect in the upper quadrants. The omental flap is very soft and can fill the partial mastectomy defect even through a small periareolar incision because of its pliability (Fig. 7.14d–f).

When the omentum is used as a free flap, the roots of the right GEAV are clipped and resected (Fig. 7.15a, b).

The omental flap is taken out from the umbilical incision or a lower abdominal incision. Anastomoses are performed between the right gastroepiploic vessels and the thoracodorsal vessels (Fig. 7.15c).

The internal thoracic vessels can also be used for recipients. After anastomoses are completed (Fig. 7.15d), the very pliable free omental flap can fill the partial mastectomy defect through a small axillary incision (Fig. 7.15e).

The omental flap also can be applied in immediate implant reconstruction, instead of acellular dermal matrix or the LD flap. NSM is undergone through an inframammary incision (Fig. 7.16a, b).

After the omental flap is harvested (Fig. 7.16c), the implant is simply placed onto the pectoralis muscle (Fig. 7.16d) and completely covered with the omental flap (Fig. 7.16e). Figure 7.16f–i illustrate the postoperative results.

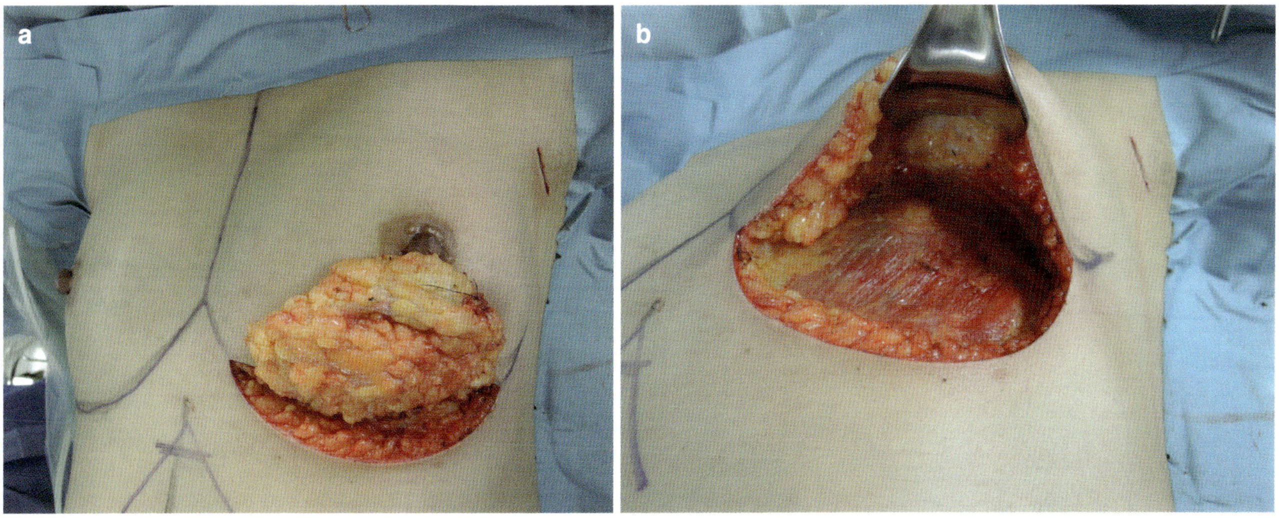

Fig. 7.7 (**a**, **b**) Partial mastectomy with an inframammary incision is the preferable choice for the omental flap to reconstruct a partial mastectomy defect in the lower quadrants

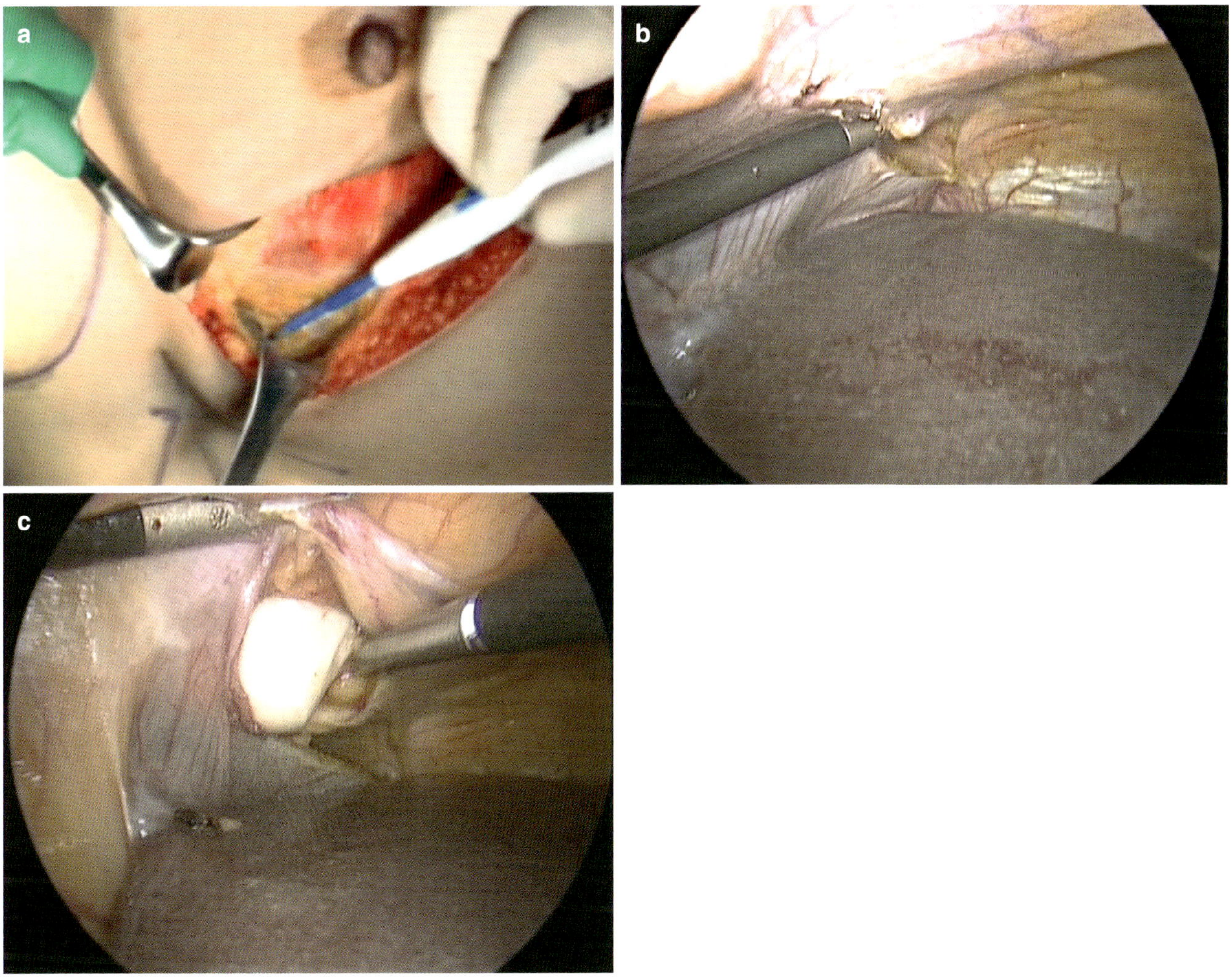

Fig. 7.8 (**a**) A subcutaneous tunnel is created from the medial site of the skin incision toward the xiphoidal process. After the tunnel reaches the white line, a longitudinal incision is made to communicate with the abdominal cavity. (**b**) Intra-abdominal resection of the peritoneum. (**c**) An incision 2–2.5 fingerbreadths wide is required to extract the omental flap

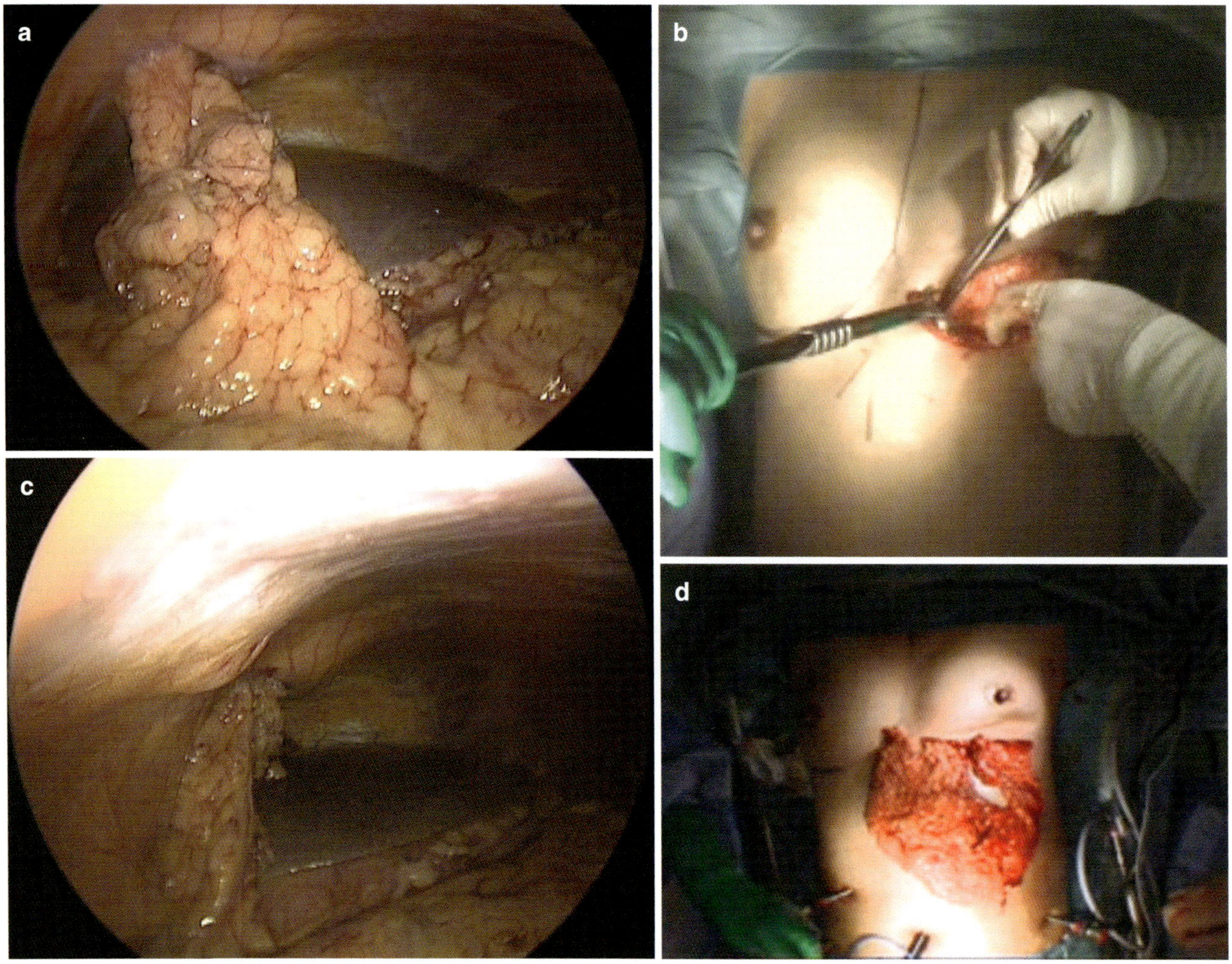

Fig. 7.9 (**a**) The omental flap is gently pulled out of the abdominal cavity. If the volume of the flap is large, this step is difficult, and a longitudinal abdominal skin incision may be required. (**b**) The omental flap is extracted through the subcutaneous tunnel. (**c**) The pedicle of the flap should be as thin as possible to prevent bulging of the subcutaneous tunnel. (**d**) The pedicled omental flap

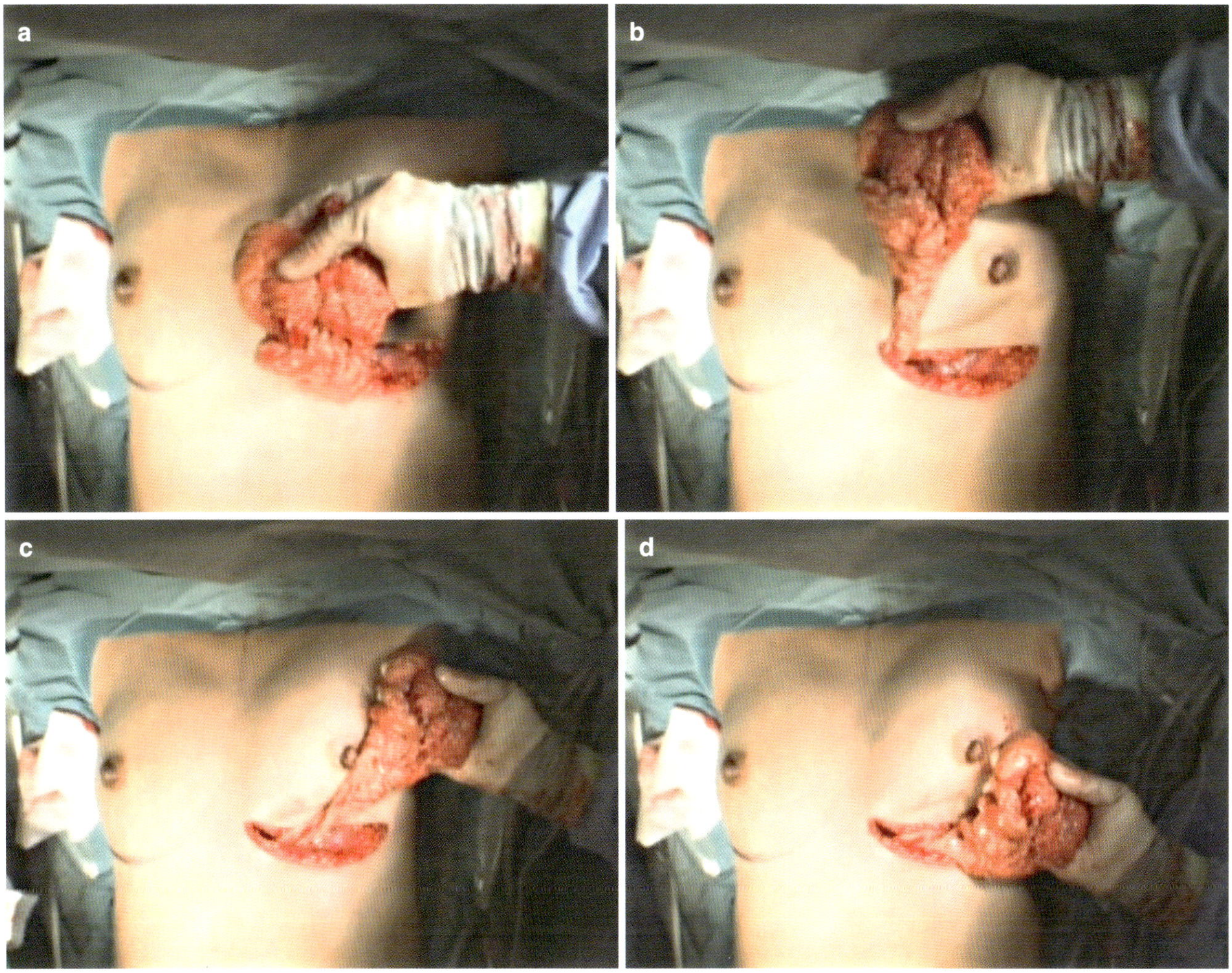

Fig. 7.10 (**a**–**d**) The omental flap can reach any quadrants of the breast. Volume replacements for the medial quadrants (**a**, **b**) are difficult with other autologous flaps but are a comfortable field for the omental flap

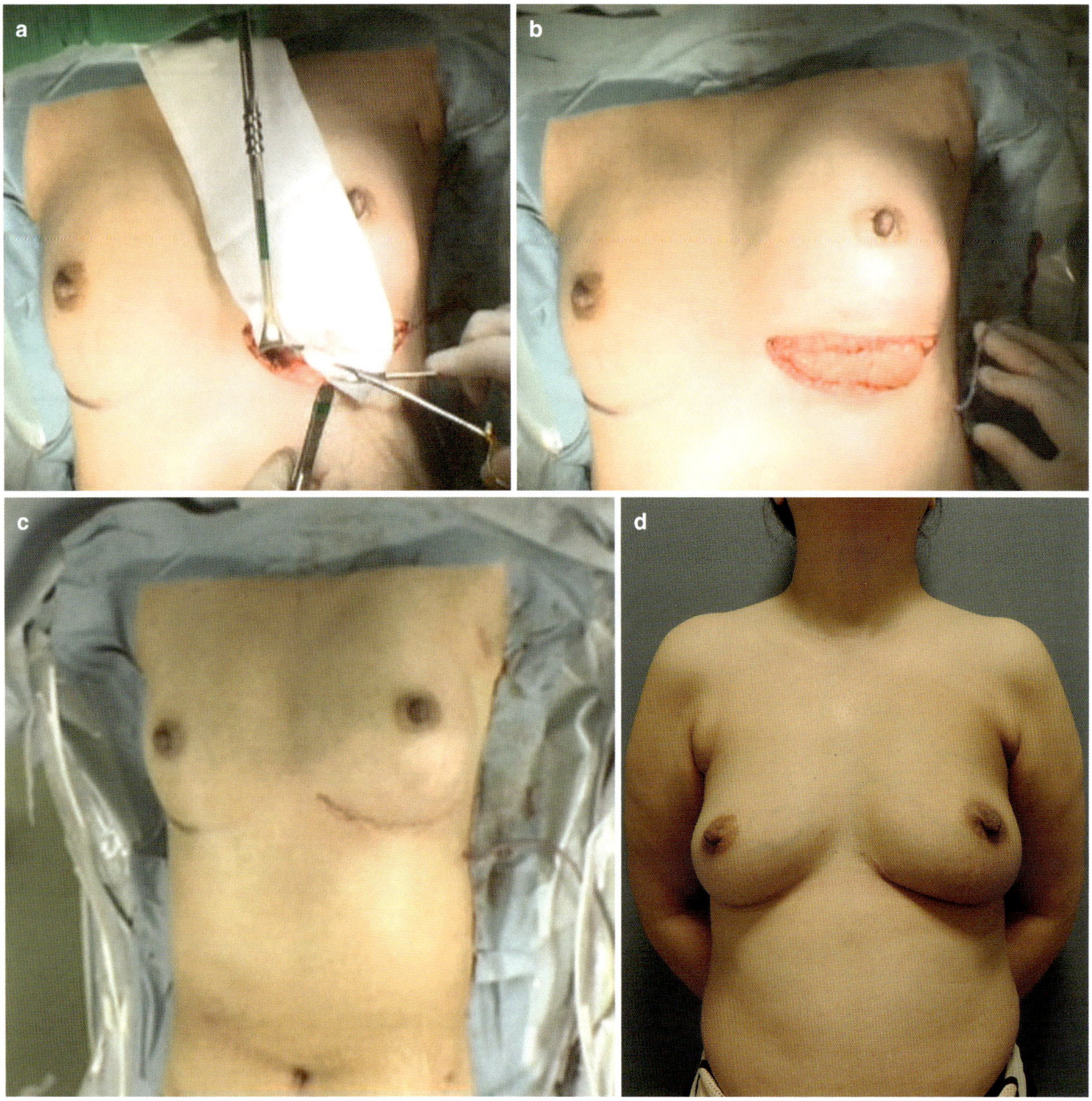

Fig. 7.11 (**a**) The subcutaneous tunnel is semi-closed to be less than 2 cm in width. (**b**) Fixation of the omental flap is usually unnecessary. (**c**) Donor-site scars are negligible. (**d**, **e**) One year after postoperative radiotherapy, this patient's reconstructed breast has a natural appearance and very soft tactile feeling

Fig. 7.12 (**a**) Partial mastectomy including the left lower inner quadrant was performed with an inframammary incision. (**b**) The omental flap was extracted through the same incision. (**c**) Three years after postoperative and radiotherapy

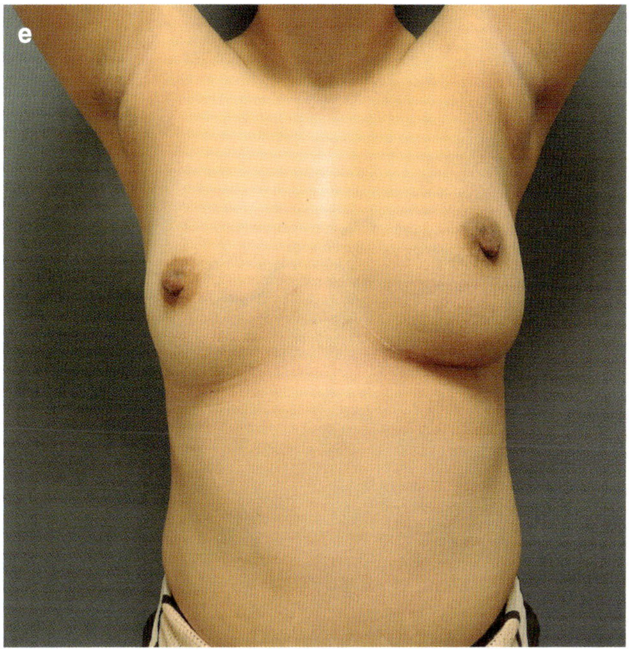

Fig. 7.11 (continued)

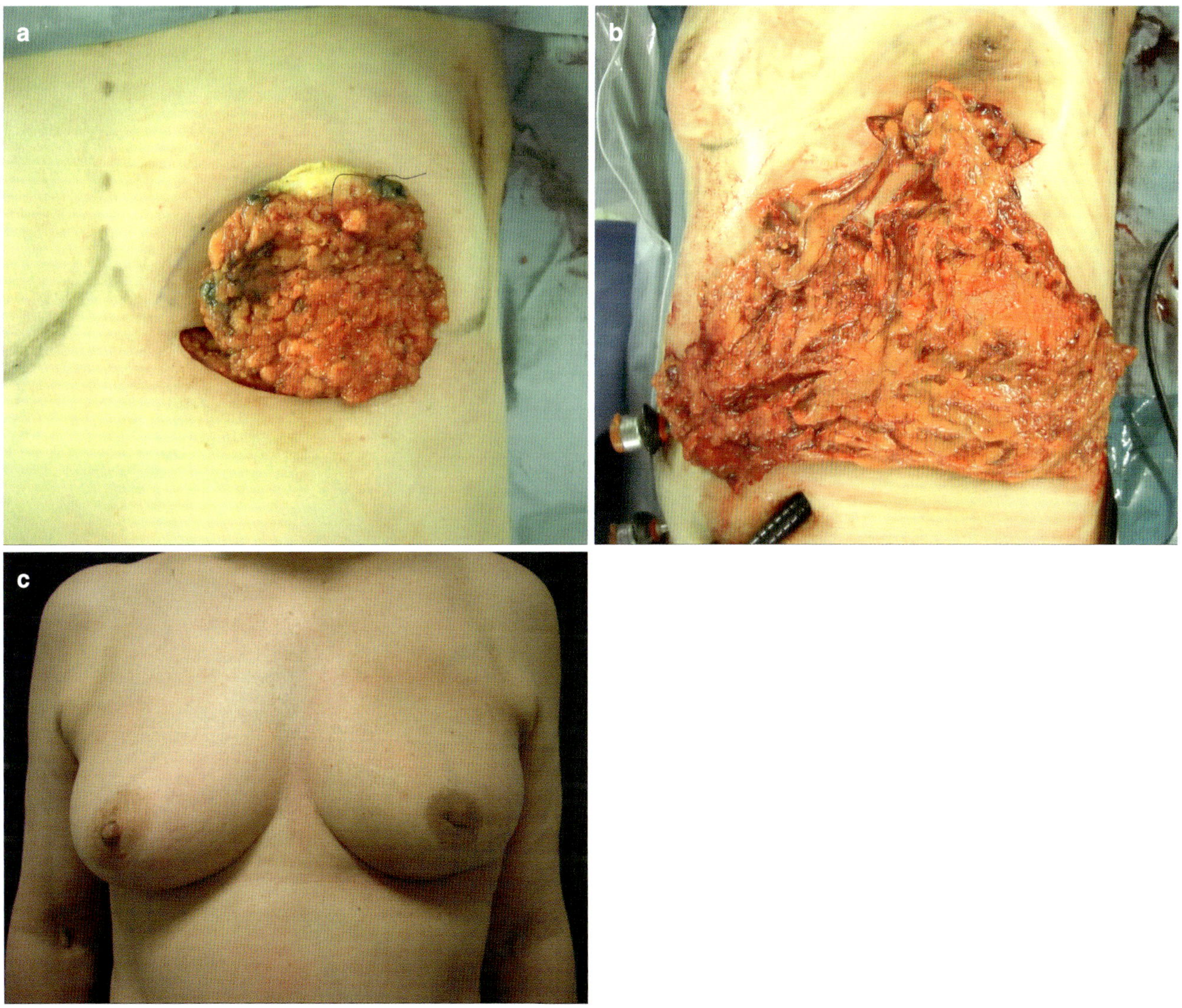

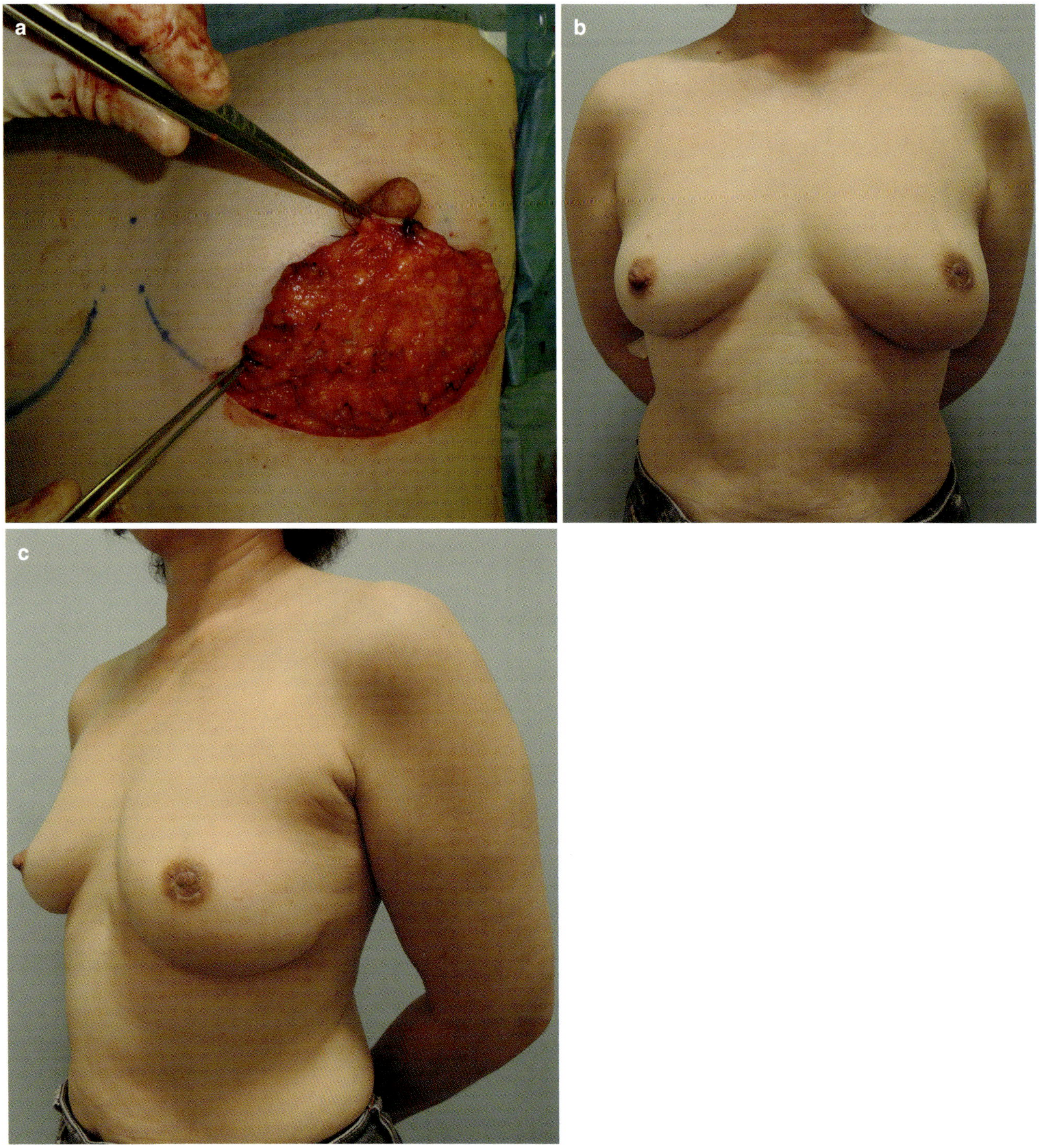

Fig. 7.13 (**a**) Partial mastectomy with an inframammary incision for a tumor in the lower central location. (**b**, **c**) One year after immediate partial reconstruction with the omental flap. Postoperative radiotherapy was also added

Fig. 7.14 (**a**) Partial mastectomy including the whole upper inner quadrant was performed with a periareolar incision. (**b**) A small incision was made on the medial inframammary fold and the omental flap was extracted through the subcutaneous tunnel. (**c**) One year after postoperative radiotherapy. (**d**) Partial mastectomy was performed with radial incision to resect the skin overlying the tumor. (**e**) A small incision was made on the medial inframammary fold and the omental flap was extracted through the subcutaneous tunnel. (**f**) Three years after surgery

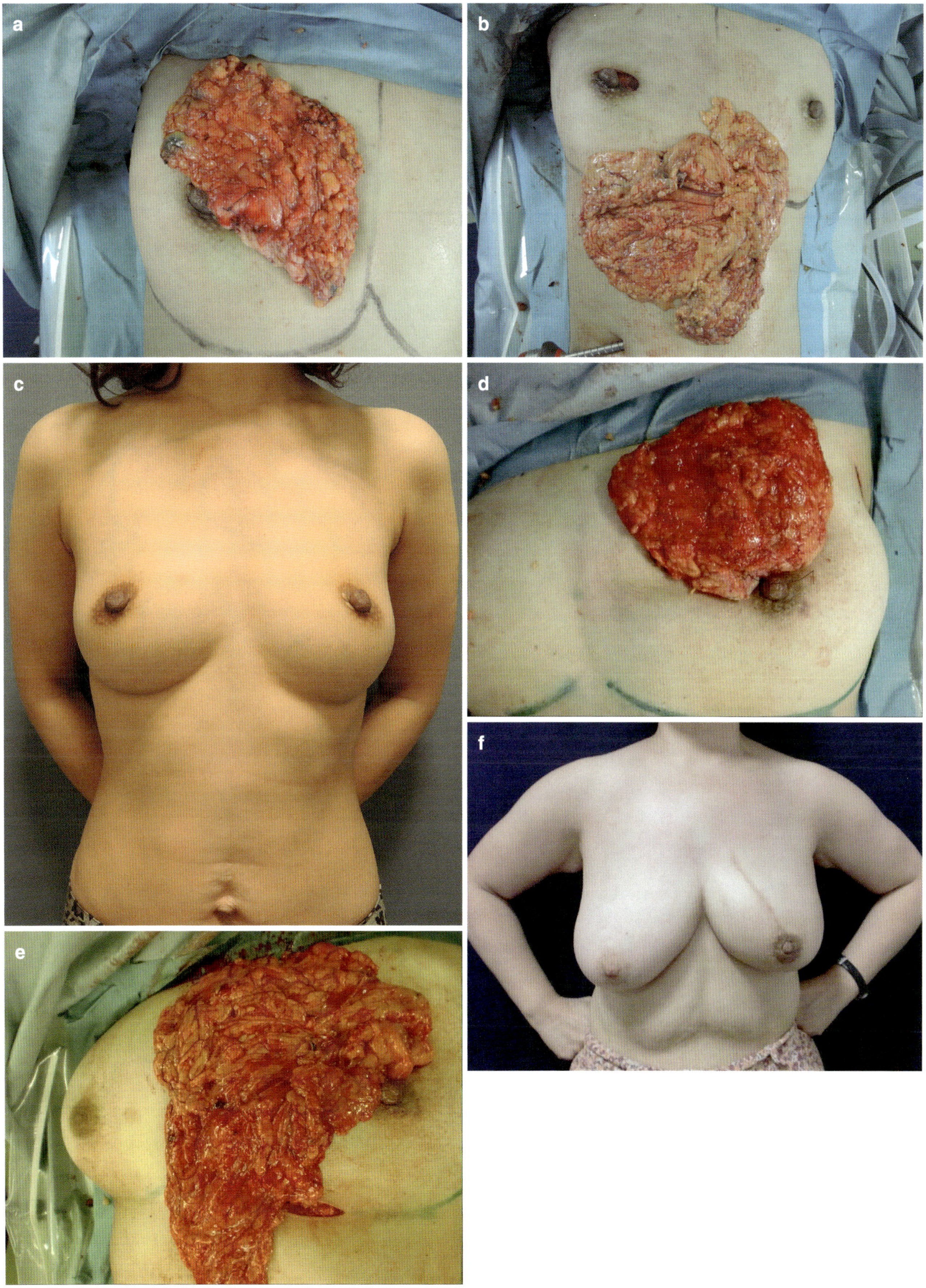
a
b
c
d
e
f

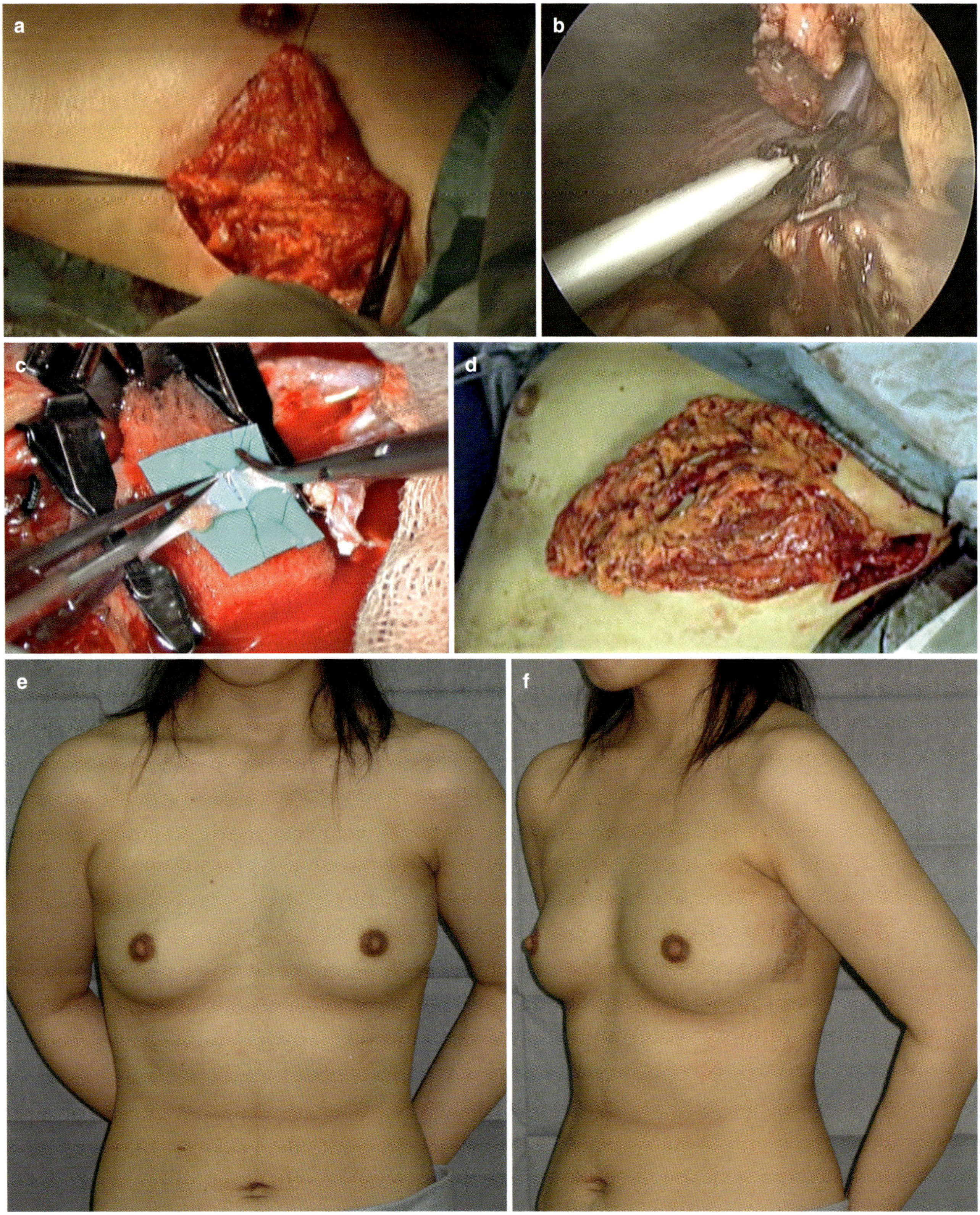

Fig. 7.15 (**a**) Partial mastectomy was performed with an anterior axillary incision. (**b**) After harvesting the omental flap, the roots of the right gastroepiploic vessels were clipped and resected. A small incision was made in the left lower abdominal wall, and the omental flap was taken out. (**c**) Anastomoses are performed between the right gastroepiploic vessels and the thoracodorsal vessels. (**d**) After the anastomoses are completed, the free omental flap is able to fill the partial mastectomy defect through a small axillary incision, because of its pliability. (**e**, **f**) Postoperative result

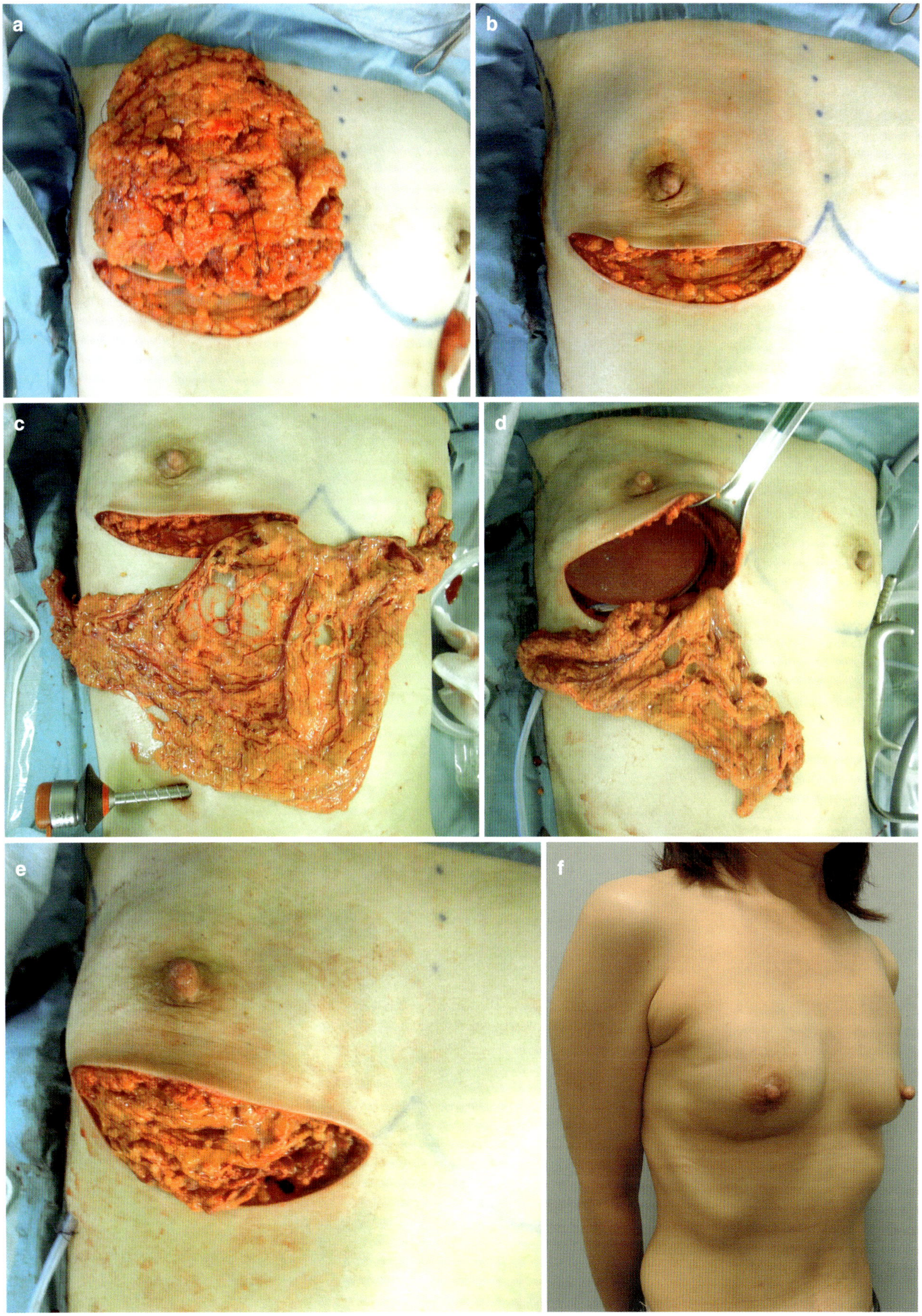

Fig. 7.16 (**a**, **b**) Nipple-sparing mastectomy was performed with an inframammary incision. (**c**) The omental flap was harvested and extracted through the subcutaneous tunnel. (**d**) An implant was placed onto the pectoralis muscle. (**e**) The omental flap covered the implant, and immediate reconstruction was completed. (**f–h**) Cosmetic result was very good, with very natural, soft tactile feeling. (**i**) Postoperative MRI showed that the implant was covered with well- vascularized omental flap, and there was enough thickness between the implant and the skin

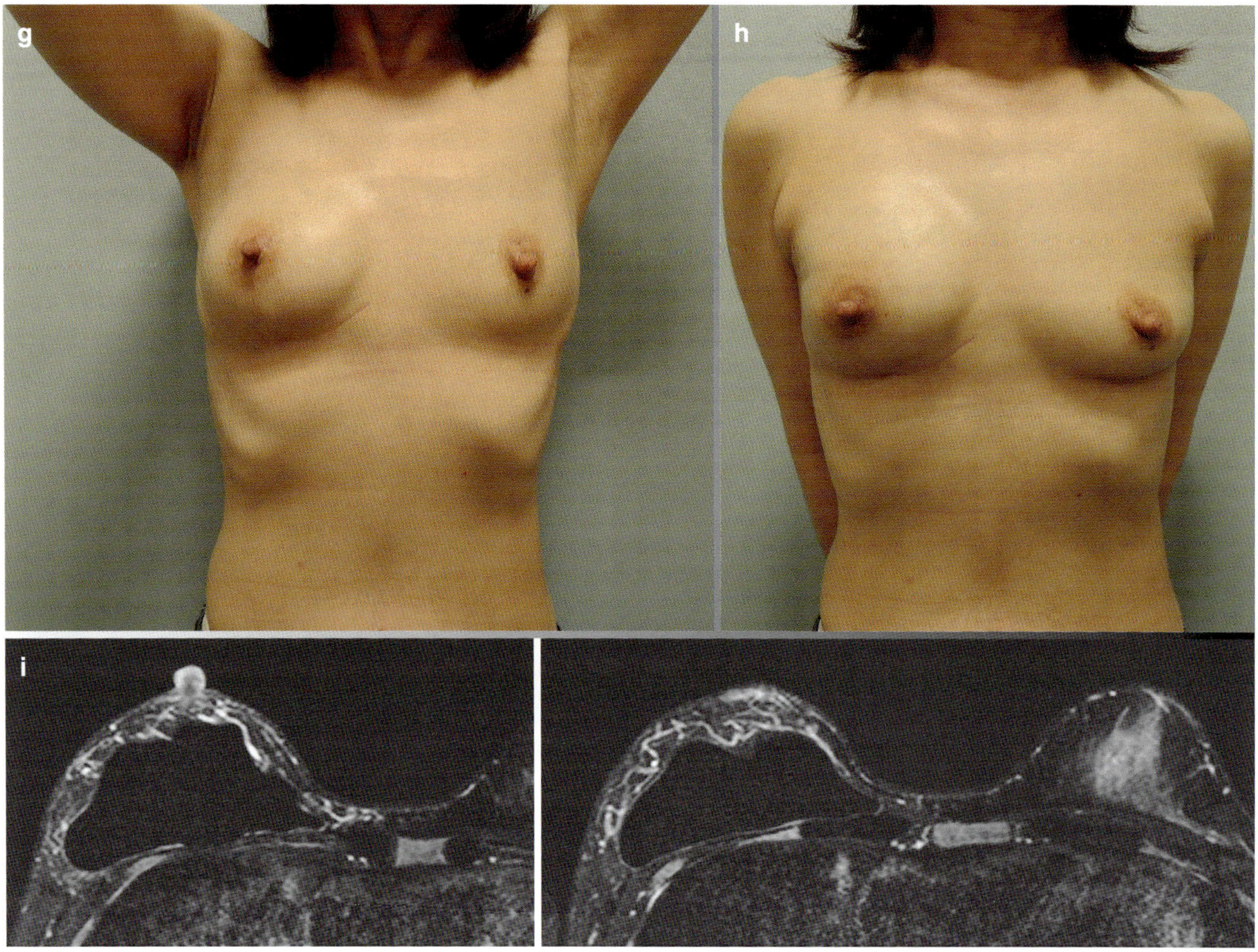

Fig. 7.16 (continued)

Conclusions

The omental flap has three main advantages:

- Minimal donor-site deformity and morbidity
- Applicability to any quadrant of the breast, especially the medial quadrants
- Softness and strength against radiation therapy

In our series of 96 patients [6], the omental flaps were successfully harvested in 99 % of the patients without conversion to open surgery. Laparoscopy-associated complications occurred in only 3.1 %, including vascular injury of the gastroepiploic artery (2.1 %) and incisional hernia (1.0 %). Small bowel obstruction did not occur. Partial graft necrosis occurred in 5.2 % of patients and was treated conservatively in all cases. The degree of donor-site scars was similar to that of laparoscopic cholecystectomy, and postoperative recovery was fast.

Recent advances in the use of a lateral chest wall perforator flap such as the TDAP and the LICAP flaps also can minimize donor-site morbidity and deformity, but their use leaves a scar on the lateral chest wall.

In partial reconstruction, the medial quadrants are distant and difficult for the other autologous flaps, but close and easy for the omental flap. Placing an invisible incision along the inframammary fold affords excellent access to the abdominal cavity. The partial mastectomy defect can be filled even through a small incision because of the pliability of the omental flap.

The main disadvantage of the omental flap is that preoperative estimation of the omental volume is not possible and the volume may be insufficient. Insufficient volume is rarely a problem for cases of partial reconstruction, but care must be taken when the breast to be reconstructed is large. On the other hand, when the omental volume is large enough for total reconstruction, it is difficult to withdraw the omental flap via the subcutaneous tunnel without adding a longitudinal abdominal incision. In such cases, a free omental flap is a better choice, because any large, free omental flaps can be easily extracted through a small but flexible lower abdominal incision.

Another advantage of the omental flap is that it usually undergoes less atrophy (even after radiation therapy) than a muscle flap, and it is softer than other autologous flaps.

This use of the laparoscopically harvested omental flap thus provides an additional option for partial breast reconstruction.

References

1. Kiricuta I. L'emploi du grand epiploon dans la chirurgie du sein cancereux. Presse Med. 1963;71:15–7.
2. Goldsmith HS. The omentum: research and clinical applications. New York: Springer; 1990.
3. Salz R, Stowers R, Smith M, Gadacz TR. Laparoscopically harvested omental free flap to cover a large soft tissue defect. Ann Surg. 1993;217:542–6.
4. Munhoz AM, Montag E, Fels KW, Arruda EG, Sturtz GP, Aldrighi C, et al. Outcome analysis of breast-conservation surgery and immediate latissimus dorsi flap reconstruction in patients with T1 to T2 breast cancer. Plast Reconstr Surg. 2005;116:741–52.
5. Hamdi M, Landuyt KV, Monstrey S, Blondeel P. Pedicled perforator flaps in breast reconstruction: a new concept. Br J Plast Surg. 2004;57:531–9.
6. Zaha H, Inamine S. Laparoscopically harvested omental flap: results for 96 patients. Surg Endosc. 2010;24:103–7.
7. Zaha H, Inamine S, Naito T, Nomura H. Laparoscopically harvested omental flap for immediate breast reconstruction. Am J Surg. 2006;192:556–8.
8. Zaha H, Sunagawa H, Kawakami K, Touyama T, Yonaha T, Ohshiro N. Partial breast reconstruction for an inferomedial breast carcinoma using an omental flap. World J Surg. 2010;34:1782–7.

8 Video-Assisted Thoracoscopic Sympathicotomies for the Treatment of Palmar and Axillary Hyperhidrosis

Edoardo Raposio and Giorgia Caruana

Hyperhidrosis of the upper limbs is a relatively common functional disorder (1–3 % prevalence) [1] that may negatively impact patients' daily activities and quality of life, with social and occupational challenges. The prevalence and embarrassing nature of this disorder has roused the interest of many [2–10], but significant controversies still surround surgical treatments of primary hyperhidrosis.

Conservative treatments such as topical aluminum chloride hexahydrate, anticholinergic drugs, iontophoresis, or injection of botulinum toxin have proved to be only partially useful for a short time [11]. Similarly, alcohol block of the sympathetic chain is unsatisfactory, as the effect is unpredictable and usually not permanent [12].

Various surgical methods of destroying axillary sweat glands by local excision have been described [13–18]. The complications of these procedures include wound infection, skin flap necrosis, and prominent, ugly scars that may be associated with marked contracture that impairs arm mobility.

Among the large spectrum of treatments suggested over the years, a video-assisted thoracoscopic approach is now widely recommended as the treatment of choice for upper limb hyperhidrosis, allowing patients to achieve a permanent solution [1, 19].

Two different endoscopic procedures are described in the literature [5, 20]: sympathicotomy (electrocautery) and sympathectomy (excision). The principle of both procedures is to interrupt the cholinergic sympathetic innervation to the eccrine glands. When the goal is treating palmar hyperhidrosis, the second (T2) and third (T3) thoracic sympathetic ganglia are interrupted; interruption of the fourth (T4) thoracic sympathetic ganglion is added when also treating axillary hyperhidrosis. Some authors [21] shared a concern about possible neural regeneration with recurrence of symptoms when sympathicotomy was performed instead of sympathectomy, but data from other authors [2, 5] showed no recurrence at all during the follow-up period, proving that recurrence after sympathicotomy might be a matter of technique. Furthermore, sympathicotomy is a rapid (mean 12 min) and less invasive procedure [2].

In 1977, Kux [22] was the first author to describe the technique of endoscopic, transthoracic upper dorsal sympathectomy for hyperhidrosis. This therapeutic approach was intended for use in patients with palmar and axillary hyperhidrosis, upper extremity ischemia (due to Raynaud's disease, for example), and upper extremity causalgia. Originally, this method relied (at least) on double trocar insertion per side, carbon dioxide insufflation, or both [22–26]. Thus, although this approach carried with it few postoperative complications when compared with traditional "open" sympathectomy techniques, it still produced some postoperative discomfort and risk of complications related to carbon dioxide insufflation, including postoperative subcutaneous emphysema and intraoperative profound bradycardia and hypotension due to mediastinal shift.

In 1995, Raposio et al. [2], in an effort to reduce the drawbacks associated with the current endoscopic techniques, introduced a minimally invasive, endoscopic, transthoracic sympathicotomy technique. The new technique is performed using a single-entry, specifically modified thoracoscope and does not require carbon dioxide insufflation.

As illustrated below, the procedure is performed under general anesthesia with a double-lumen endotracheal tube. The patient is placed in a half-sitting position, with both arms abducted to 90°. In this Raposio approach [2, 27], a 1-cm stab incision is performed, along either the mid-clavicular

E. Raposio, MD, PhD, FICS (✉)
Plastic Surgery Section, Department of Surgical Sciences, University of Parma, Via Gramsci 14, Parma 43126, Italy
e-mail: edoardo.raposio@unipr.it

G. Caruana, MD
Department of Surgical Science, Plastic Surgery Section, Parma University Hospital, Via Gramsci 14, Parma 43126, Italy
e-mail: giorgia.caruana@gmail.com

E. Raposio (ed.), *Atlas of Endoscopic Plastic Surgery*, DOI 10.1007/978-3-319-19461-5_8

line (male patients) or the anterior axillary line (female patients), in the third intercostal space. After selective deflation of the ipsilateral lung, trocar insertion, and creation of an artificial apical pneumothorax, a specifically designed thoracoscope is inserted. The dorsal sympathetic chain is visualized through the parietal pleura as it passes over the neck of the ribs close to the costovertebral junction. If simple pleural adhesions precluding access to the ganglia are encountered, they can easily be divided endoscopically. The T2, T3, and/or T4 ganglia are then severed, under direct vision, by means of the electrocautery. Special care is taken not to injure the crossing vessels in the intercostal spaces. The surgical procedure is completed by re-insufflation of the collapsed lung, insertion of a chest drain through the same operative incision, and closure of the wound with cutaneous sutures. The entire procedure is then repeated on the opposite side.

A postoperative pulmonary radiograph is routinely performed 2 h after the completion of the procedure to check for the presence of pneumothorax, hemothorax, or both.

8.1 Indications and Preoperative Consultation

Ideal candidates for thoracoscopic sympathicotomy are men and women in good health, between 18 and 65 years of age, who claim that they do not usually sweat during the night and that their symptoms started at an early age. These patients' symptoms usually appear at puberty but may date back to early childhood, and they usually persist throughout adult life [2]. Patients with a body mass index (BMI) greater than 28 and/or with other overt diseases should not be enrolled for surgery.

Surgical consultation before surgery should confirm the presence of primary focal palmar and/or axillary hyperhidrosis, the anatomic locations involved, and the amount of hyperhidrosis itself [1]. Patients should then be informed about possible risks and complications, as well as about the percentage of success or failure and the reasons for possible failure. The main reasons that may lead to an unsuccessful treatment are massive pleural adhesions, overlying vascular bundles, or thick overlying subpleural fat that obscures the sympathetic chain, thus precluding access to the ganglia and partial or total completion of the procedure.

8.2 Complications

As the main purpose of this treatment is to improve the patient's quality of life, achieving the lowest possible rate of intraoperative and postoperative complications should be central. Nevertheless, postoperative effects such as compensatory hyperhidrosis (CH), bradycardia, and Horner's syndrome are possible following video-assisted thoracoscopic selective sympathicotomy.

CH is the most common adverse effect overall, occurring in 3–98 % of patients [28]. It consists of an excess of secondary sweating, primarily affecting the trunk and the lower extremities, which, by definition, was not present in the patient before the surgery. In general, the lower the level of blockade on the chain, the higher the expected CH rate [4, 29], so patients who undergo T2–T4 video-assisted thoracoscopic electrocauterization for palmar and axillary hyperhidrosis should be made aware of the much greater likelihood of CH compared with patients who undergo only T2–T3 electrocauterization (mainly for palmar hyperhidrosis). Luckily, even though CH is perceived as discomfort by patients, most of them find the CH less burdensome than their initial palmar and/or axillary hyperhidrosis, and they usually say that they would have the procedure again [4, 10].

Permanent bradycardia also has been reported after surgery [1, 30]; it is particularly dangerous for patients who had a resting heart rate before surgery of 50–55 beats per minute. These patients may require a pacemaker, so such patients should not be enrolled for surgery.

Horner syndrome is another adverse effect, occurring in 0.7–3 % of patients [1]. It may occur when the stellate ganglion is manipulated during the surgical procedure, so it is more frequent when operating on facial hyperhidrosis, owing to improper localization of the second rib.

Less frequent complications (<1 %) that may occur after thoracoscopic sympathicotomy are pneumothorax, hemothorax, chylothorax, and infection of the incision site [1].

8.3 Surgical Technique

Figures 8.1, 8.2, 8.3, 8.4, 8.5, 8.6, 8.7, 8.8, 8.9, 8.10, 8.11, and 8.12 illustrate the steps of the endoscopic transthoracic sympathicotomy technique

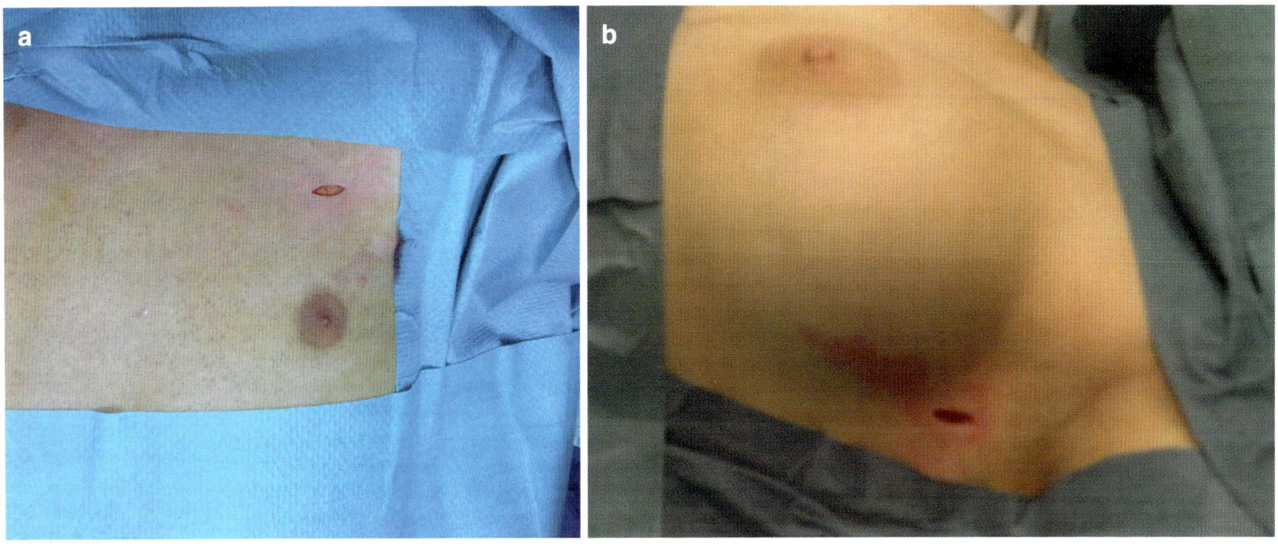

Fig. 8.1 After general anesthesia with a double-lumen endotracheal tube, the patient is placed in a half-sitting position with both arms abducted to 90°, and ribs 2 through 4 are identified. A 1-cm stab incision is then performed at third intercostal space, along the midclavicular line for male patients (**a**) and along the anterior axillary line for female patients (**b**), in order to hide the postoperative scar as much as possible

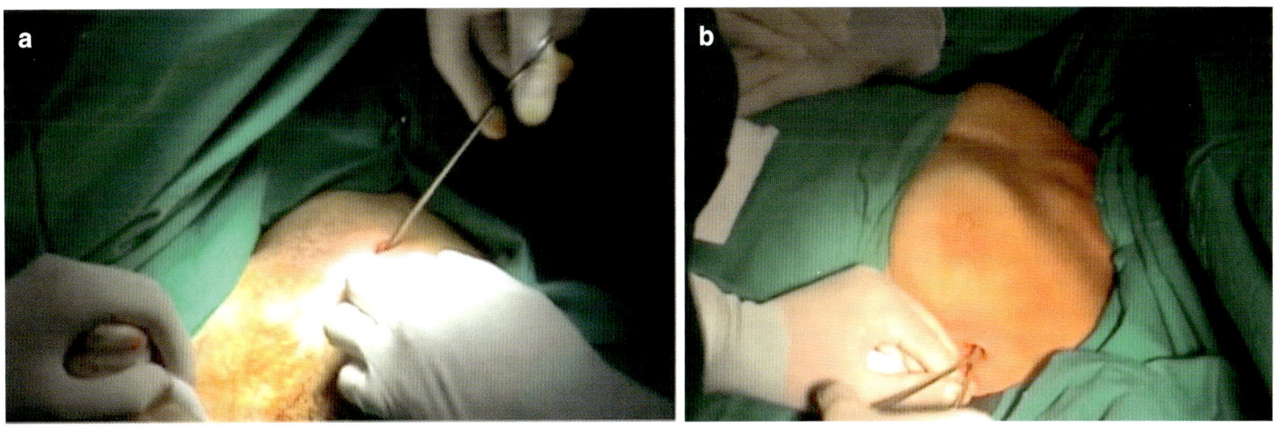

Fig. 8.2 Subcutaneous tissues are undermined through the cutaneous incision, as shown in a male (**a**) and a female (**b**) patient, in order to reach the intercostal plane at the third intercostal space. It is important during both undermining and further insertion of the endoscope that the instruments always be kept upon the upper edge of the rib, in order to avoid the neurovascular bundle located just under the surface of the lower edge of the rib

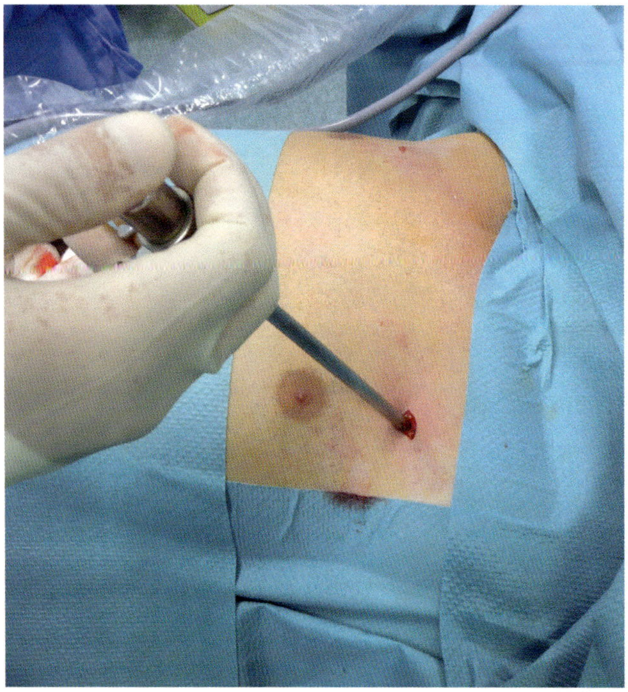

Fig. 8.3 After selective mechanical deflation and collapse of the ipsilateral lung, a 9-mm trocar with an air/insufflator/suction triple valve is inserted through the previously created incision at the third intercostal space on the left side of the patient, always keeping it on the surface of the upper edge of the rib to avoid the vascular bundle

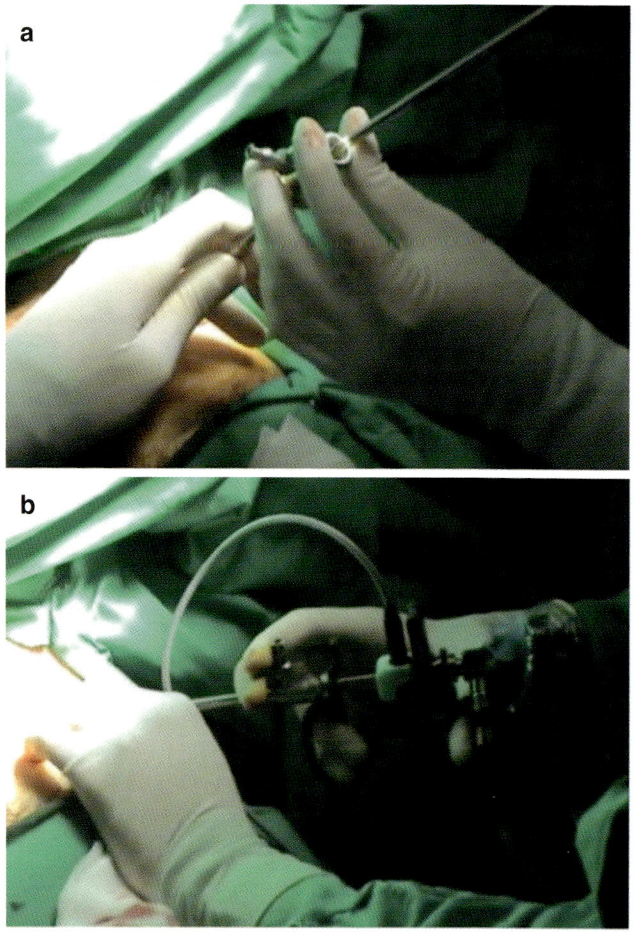

Fig. 8.4 After trocar insertion and creation of an artificial ipsilateral apical pneumothorax, a specifically designed thoracoscope (shown in Fig. 8.5) is guided through the trocar (**a**) down into the pleural cavity (**b**). From this point on, the entire procedure is displayed on the external monitor

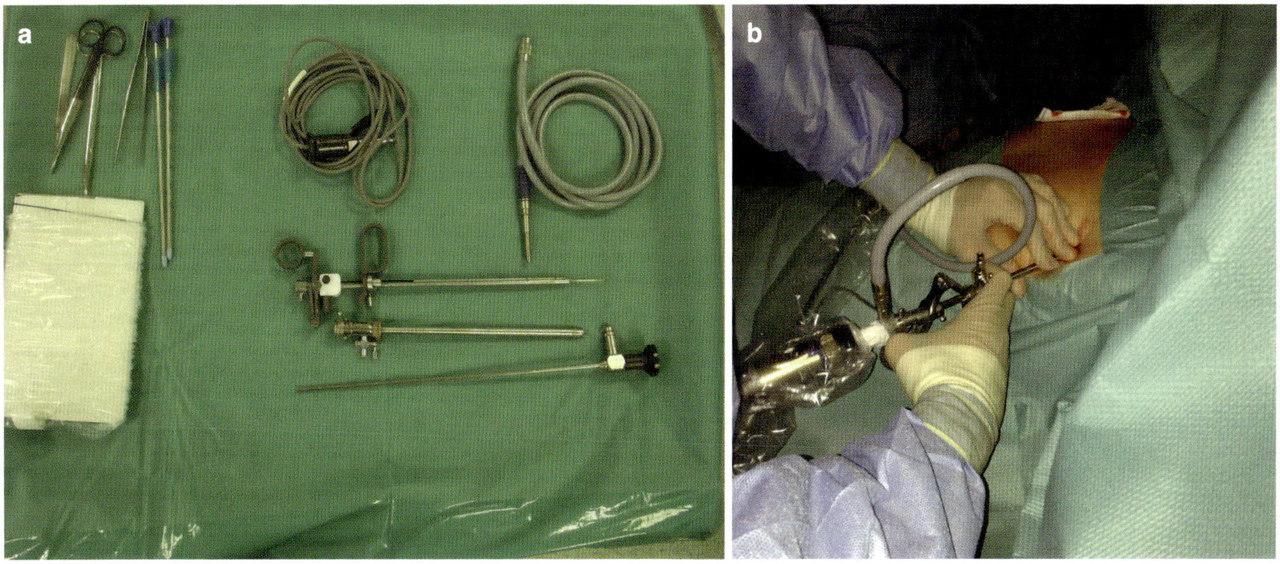

Fig. 8.5 (**a**) The modified thoracoscope (Karl Storz; Tuttlingen, Germany) consists of a 9-mm trocar with air/insufflator/suction triple valve, a straight Hopkins telescope with fiber-light transmission, a Wittmöser operating sheath with a connection for high-frequency diathermy, and a specifically designed triangle-tipped wire loop electrode for the electrocautery. (**b**) The thoracoscope enters the pleural cavity through the previously performed incision (third intercostal space) while the patient trunk is positioned at 45°

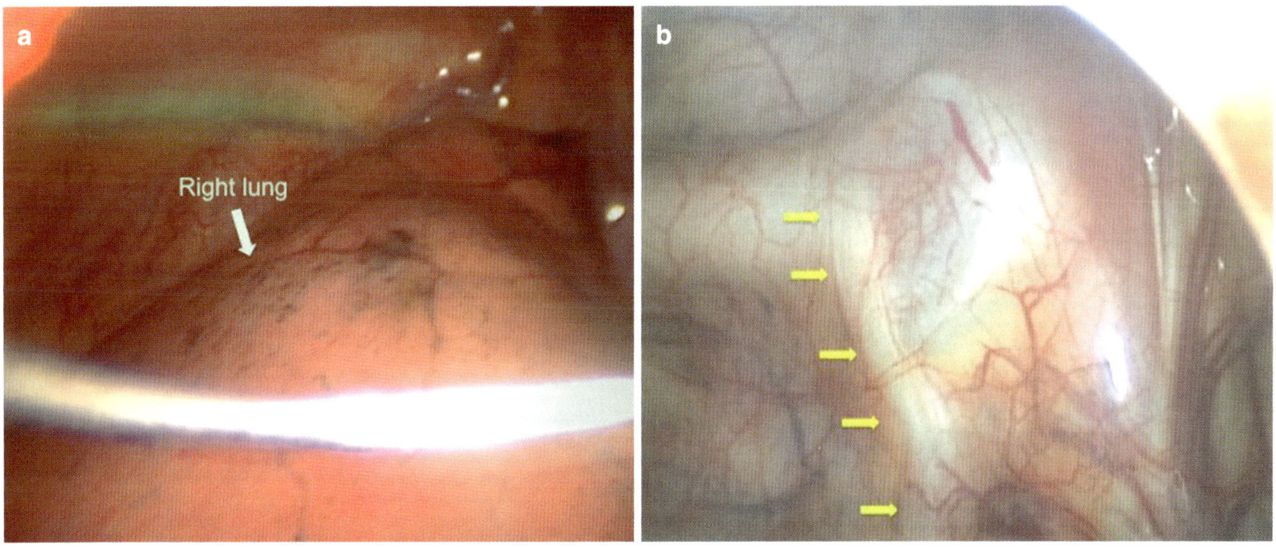

Fig. 8.6 (**a**) Following ipsilateral lung deflation, the modified thoracoscope is introduced into the thoracic cavity, where the mediastinum is now visible. (**b**) The right dorsal sympathetic chain (*yellow arrows*) is visualized through the parietal pleura as it passes over the neck of the ribs close to the costovertebral junction

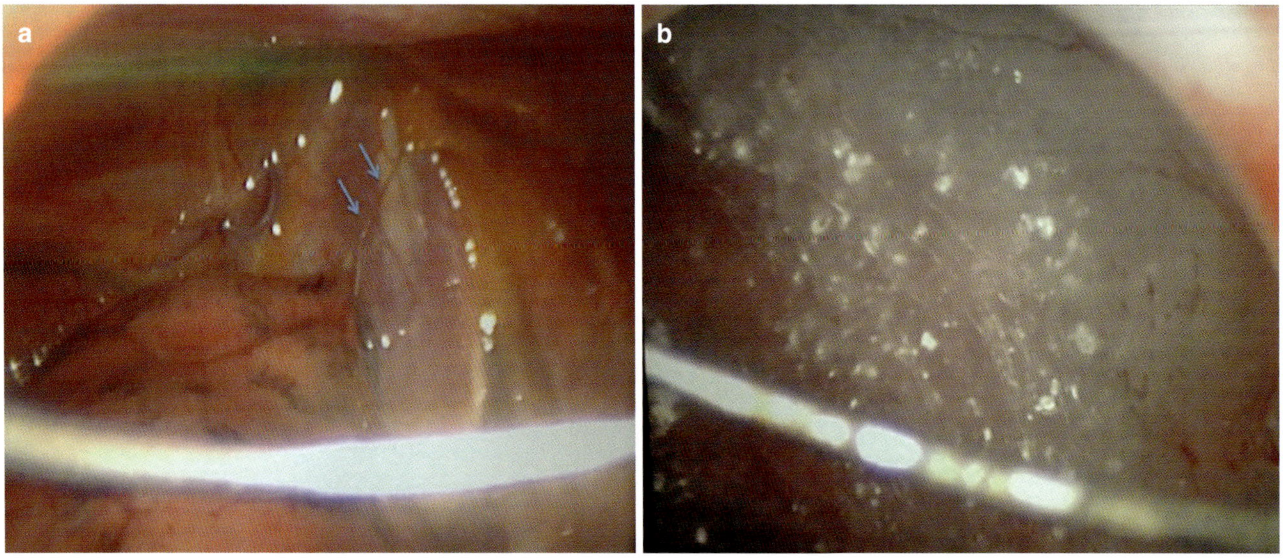

Fig. 8.7 Sometimes, small pleural adhesions (**a**, *blue arrows*) to widespread pleural adhesions (**b**) may be found, which preclude access to the ganglia and limit the completion of the procedure. If removal of the pleural adhesions is thought to be without risk, they can easily be divided endoscopically

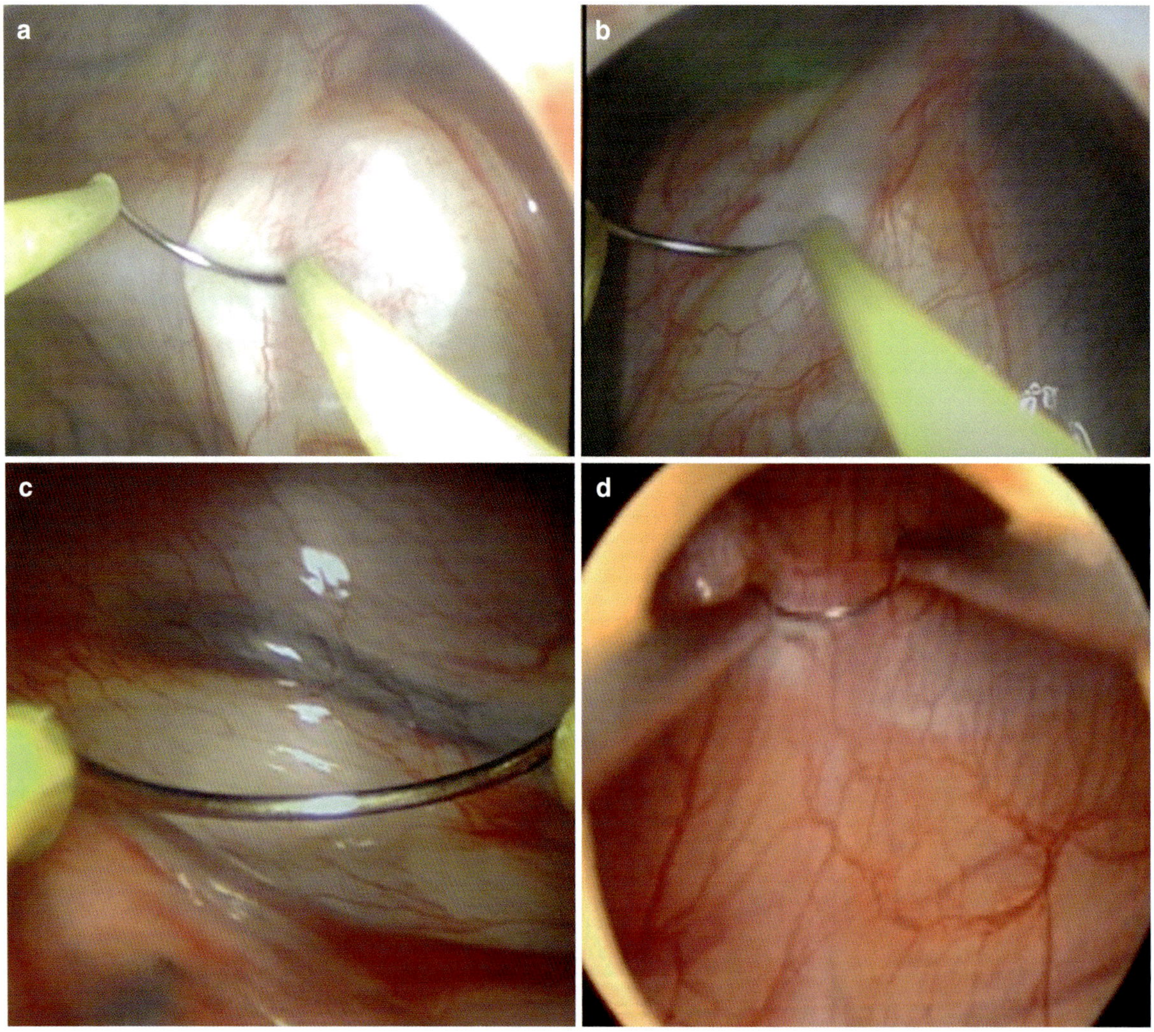

Fig. 8.8 (**a–d**) The ribs are endoscopically identified, as well as the sympathetic chain, which appears as a pink/white longitudinal structure protruding over the neck of the ribs, close to the costovertebral junction

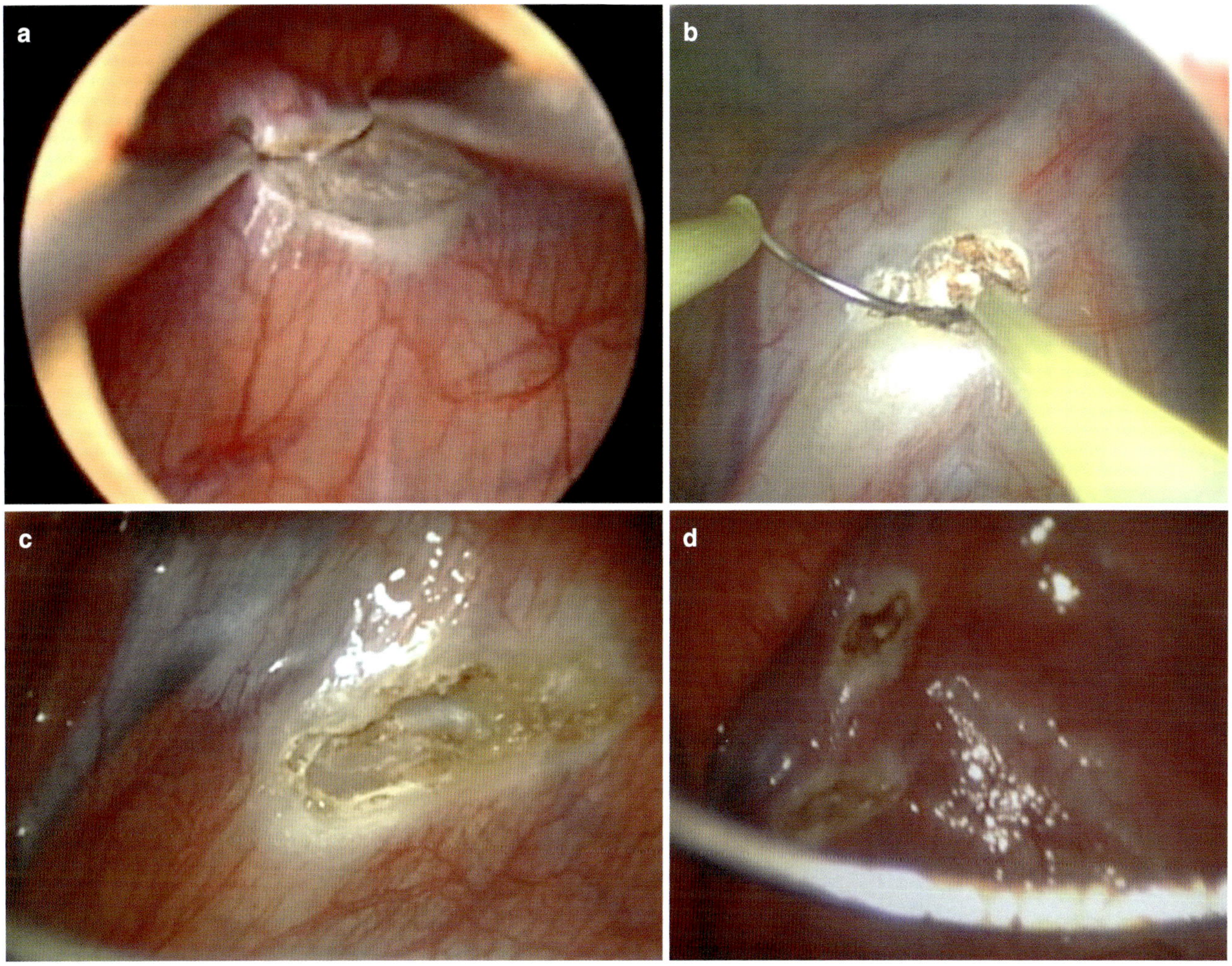

Fig. 8.9 (**a**–**d**) Electrocauterization (sympathicotomy) of the second, third, and/or fourth thoracic sympathetic ganglia (T2, T3, T4) is then performed, with special care to not injure the crossing vessels in the intercostal spaces or nearby (**c**)

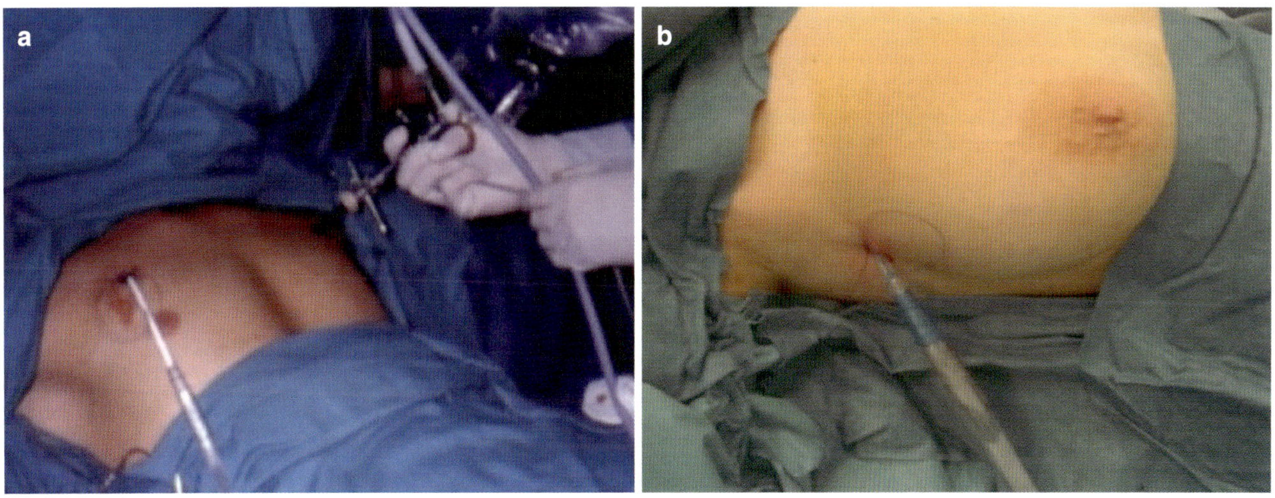

Fig. 8.10 The surgical procedure on the first side is completed by re-insufflation of the collapsed lung, insertion of a chest drain by the same operative incision on the mid-clavicular (**a**) or anterior axillary (**b**) line, and closure of the wound with cutaneous sutures. The entire procedure is then repeated on the opposite side

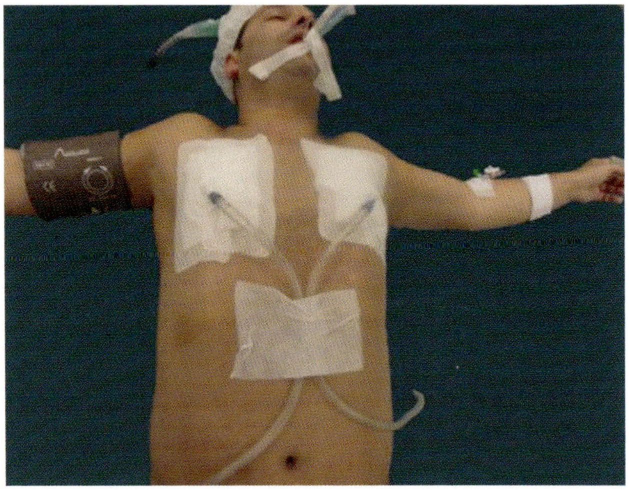

Fig. 8.11 Male patient after surgery in a half-sitting position with both arms abducted to 90°, before removal of the double-lumen endotracheal tube. Surgical dressings are applied on both sides to cover the incisions and keep the chest drains from moving

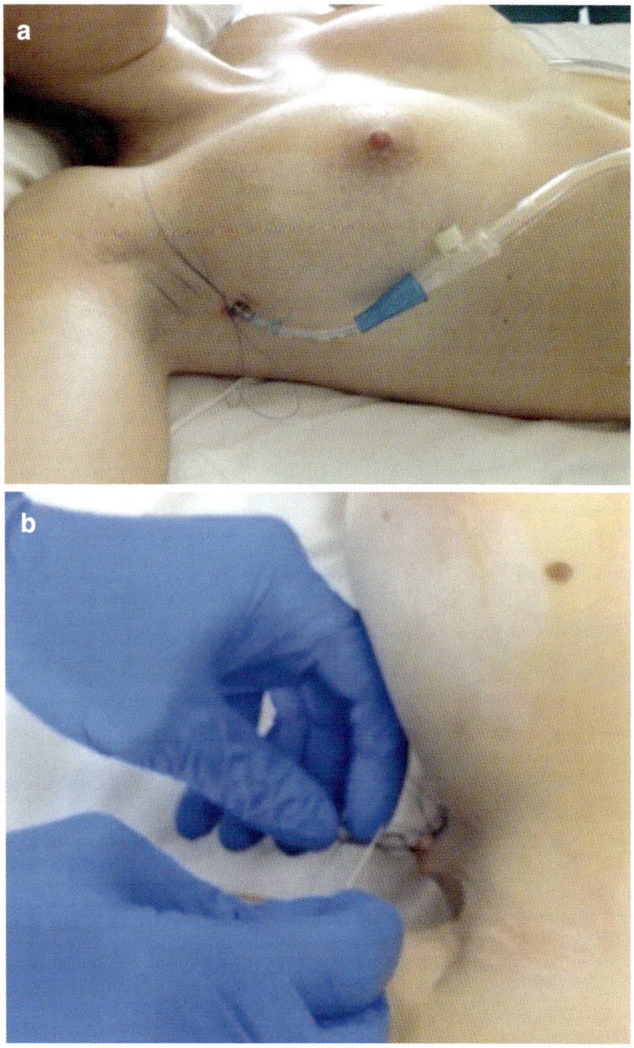

Fig. 8.12 (**a**, **b**) Removal of chest drains is performed 2 h after surgery, if a postoperative pulmonary radiograph has excluded the presence of pneumothorax or hemothorax. A #11 blade is used to cut the suture knot tied around the tube; once the knot is untied, the drain on one side is extracted from the chest with a rapid movement. Another operator then immediately ties the knot that was sutured all around the tube, in this way closing the incision

Conclusions

Minimally invasive endoscopic transthoracic sympathicotomy [2] has proven to be an effective and durable surgical treatment for severe primary hyperhidrosis. It significantly improves the quality of life of treated patients. The procedure is not only durable but also less invasive than previous approaches, and (depending on operator experience) it results in fewer postoperative complications; for example, in our experience, we have never reported one case of Horner syndrome in more than 800 patients.

References

1. Cerfolio RJ, De Campos JR, Bryant AS, Connery CP, Miller DL, DeCamp MM, et al. The Society of Thoracic Surgeons expert consensus for the surgical treatment of hyperhidrosis. Ann Thorac Surg. 2011;91:1642–8.
2. Raposio E, Filippi F, Nordström RE, Santi P. Endoscopic transthoracic dorsal sympathectomy for the treatment of upper extremity hyperhidrosis: a new minimally invasive approach. Plast Reconstr Surg. 1998;102:1629–32.
3. Ahn SS, Ro KM. Thoracoscopic sympathectomy. Ann Vasc Surg. 1998;12:509–14.
4. Riet M, Smet AA, Kuiken H, Kazemier G, Bonjer HJ. Prevention of compensatory hyperhidrosis after thoracoscopic sympathectomy for hyperhidrosis. Surg Endosc. 2001;15:1159–62.
5. Kim BY, Oh BS, Park YK, Jang WC, Suh HJ, Im YH. Microinvasive video-assisted thoracoscopic sympathicotomy for primary palmar hyperhidrosis. Am J Surg. 2001;181:540–2.
6. Lesèche G, Castier Y, Thabut G, Petit MD, Combes M, Cerceau O, Besnard M. Endoscopic transthoracic sympathectomy for upper limb hyperhidrosis: limited sympathectomy does not reduce postoperative compensatory sweating. J Vasc Surg. 2003;37:124–8.
7. Dumont P, Denoyer A, Robin P. Long-term results of thoracoscopic sympathectomy for hyperhidrosis. Ann Thorac Surg. 2004;78:1801–7.
8. Licht PB, Jørgensen OD, Ladegaard L, Pilegaard HK. Thoracoscopic sympathectomy for axillary hyperhidrosis: the influence of T4. Ann Thorac Surg. 2005;80:455–9.
9. Dewey TM, Herbert MA, Hill SL, Prince SL, Mack MJ. One-year follow-up after thoracoscopic sympathectomy for hyperhidrosis: outcomes and consequences. Ann Thorac Surg. 2006;81:1227–32.
10. Rodríguez PM, Freixinet JL, Hussein M, Valencia JM, Gil RM, Herrero J, Caballero-Hidalgo A. Side effects, complications and outcome of thoracoscopic sympathectomy for palmar and axillary hyperhidrosis in 406 patients. Eur J Cardiothorac Surg. 2008;34:514–9.
11. Karamfilov T, Konrad H, Karte K, Wollina U. Lower relapse rate of botulinum toxin a therapy for axillary hyperhidrosis by dose increase. Arch Dermatol. 2000;136:487–90.
12. White JW. Treatment of primary hyperhidrosis. Mayo Clin Proc. 1986;61:951–5.
13. Breach NM. Axillary hyperhidrosis: surgical cure with aesthetic scars. Ann R Coll Surg Engl. 1979;61:295–8.
14. Bretteville-Jensen G. Radical sweat gland ablation for axillary hyperhidrosis. Br J Plast Surg. 1973;26:158–61.
15. Hartfall WG, Jochimsen PR. Hyperhidrosis of the upper extremity and its treatment. Surg Gynecol Obstet. 1972;135:586–90.
16. Hurley HJ, Shelley WB. A simple surgical approach to the management of axillary hyperhidrosis. JAMA. 1963;186:109–12.
17. Hurley HJ, Shelley WB. Axillary hyperhidrosis: clinical features and local surgical management. Br J Dermatol. 1966;78: 127–31.
18. Stenquist B. Axillary hyperhidrosis: a simple surgical procedure. J Dermatol Surg Oncol. 1985;11:388–91.
19. Kim WO, Kil HK, Yoon KB, Yoon DM, Lee JS. Influence of T3 or T4 sympathicotomy for palmar hyperhidrosis. Am J Surg. 2010;199:166–9.
20. Scognamillo F, Serventi F, Attene F, Torre C, Paliogiannis P, Pala C, Trignano E, Trignano M. T2-T4 sympathectomy versus T3-T4 sympathicotomy for palmar and axillary hyperhidrosis. Clin Auton Res. 2011;21:97–102.
21. Collin J. Treating hyperhidrosis: surgery and botulinum toxin are treatments of choice in severe cases. BMJ. 2000;320:1221–2.
22. Kux M. Thoracic endoscopic sympathectomy for treatment of upper limb hyperhidrosis. Lancet. 1977;1:1320–3.
23. Byrne J, Walsh TN, Hederman WP. Endoscopic transthoracic electrocautery of the sympathetic chain for palmar and axillary hyperhidrosis. Br J Surg. 1990;77:1046–50.
24. Claes G, Drott C, Göthberg G. Endoscopic electrocautery of the thoracic sympathetic chain. Scand J Plast Reconstr Surg Hand Surg. 1993;27:18–21.
25. Edmondson RA, Banerjee AK, Rennie JA. Endoscopic transthoracic sympathectomy in the treatment of hyperhidrosis. Ann Surg. 1992;215:289–92.
26. Stokes MA, O'Hanlon DM, Quill DS. Trans-thoracic sympathectomy: an improved technique. Minim Invasive Ther Allied Technol. 1994;3:135–8.
27. Raposio E, Caruana G. Video-assisted thoracic sympathicotomy for the treatment of palmar and axillary hyperhidrosis: a 17-year experience. Surg Laparosc Endosc Percutan Tech. 2015. [Epub ahead of print].
28. Lyra Rde M, Campos JR, Kang DW, Loureiro Mde P, Furian MB, Costa MG, Coelho Mde S. Sociedade Brasileira de Cirurgia Torácica. Guidelines for the prevention, diagnosis and treatment of compensatory hyperhidrosis. J Bras Pneumol. 2008;34: 967–77.
29. Chou SH, Kao EL, Lin CC, Chang YT, Huang MF. The importance of classification in sympathetic surgery and a proposed mechanism for compensatory hyperhidrosis: experience with 464 cases. Surg Endosc. 2006;20:1749–53.
30. Lay CL, Chen WJ, Liu YB, Lee YT. Bradycardia and permanent pacing after bilateral thoracoscopic T2-sympathectomy for primary hyperhidrosis. Pacing Clin Electrophysiol. 2001;24: 524–5.

Endoscopic Diastasis Recti Repair

9

Manash Ranjan Sahoo

Rectus abdominis diastasis (or diastasis recti) is mainly an acquired condition with clinically evident separation of the rectus abdominis muscle pillars. The result is a characteristic bulging of the abdominal wall that is sometimes mistaken for a ventral hernia despite the fact that the midline aponeurosis is intact and no hernia defect is present. This condition has no associated mortality or morbidity other than cosmetic concerns.

Diastasis may be congenital, as a result of a more lateral insertion of the rectus muscles to the ribs and costochondral junctions, but more typically it is an acquired condition, occurring with advancing age, in obesity, or after pregnancy. In the postpartum setting, rectus diastasis tends to occur in women with advanced maternal age, a twin or multiple pregnancy, or delivery of a high-birth-weight infant. Diastasis is usually easily identified on physical examination. CT scanning provides an accurate means of measuring the distance between the rectus pillars and can differentiate rectus diastasis from a true ventral hernia if clarification is required.

Surgical correction of rectus diastasis by plication of the broad midline aponeurosis has been described for cosmetic indications and for alleviation of impaired abdominal wall muscular function. These approaches introduce the risk of an actual ventral hernia, however, and are of questionable value in addressing pathology [1–11].

There are no current guidelines on the treatment of diastasis recti. Open divarication repair is not very popular because of associated morbidity and cosmetically unacceptable results. More recently, various surgeons have attempted to reduce the morbidity and length of scar associated with conventional open procedures. Laparoscopic repair of diastasis recti has seldom been described in literature [7, 12].

Diastasis recti may appear as a ridge running down the midline of the abdomen, anywhere from the xiphoid process to the umbilicus. It becomes more prominent with straining and may disappear when the abdominal muscles are relaxed. It is more common in multiparous women, owing to repeated episodes of stretching. The condition must be differentiated from an epigastric hernia or an incisional hernia, if the patient has had abdominal surgery. Hernias may be ruled out using ultrasound.

In some adults, diastasis recti can be corrected or mitigated by physiotherapy. A study conducted at the Columbia University Program in Physical Therapy established that the women utilizing the Tupler Technique exercises had a smaller diastasis than the control group who did not do these exercises [13]. Operative repair for diastasis recti remains controversial; few studies have assessed the effectiveness of surgical intervention. It is usually the patients themselves who request treatment. In extreme cases, diastasis recti is corrected during the cosmetic surgery procedure known as a "tummy tuck" by creating a plication or folding of the linea alba and suturing together.

9.1 Indications, Contraindications, and Preoperative Assessment

Indications for endoscopic diastasis recti repair include cosmetic disfigurement and pain. The only absolute contraindication is the inability to undergo general anaesthesia; relative contraindications include chronic obstructive pulmonary disease (COPD), morbid obesity, and cardiac morbidities.

Preoperative confirmation of the diagnosis is done by ultrasonogram, CT, and MRI. Routine hematological, biochemical, cardiac, and pulmonary assessments are also performed.

M.R. Sahoo, MS, FAIS, FMAS, FALS
Department of Surgery, Sriram Chandra Bhanj Medical College, Cuttack, Odisha 753007, India
e-mail: manash67@gmail.com

E. Raposio (ed.), *Atlas of Endoscopic Plastic Surgery*, DOI 10.1007/978-3-319-19461-5_9

9.2 Surgical Technique

The patient is put under general anesthesia for diagnostic laparoscopy. The defect is made prominent by compression from the outside and the size is assessed (Figs. 9.1, 9.2, 9.3, and 9.4).

A 48-mm needle with double loop 1 (4 metric) 48 mm ½ circle heavy round bodied Ethilon (monofilament polyamide black) (Ethicon; Somerville, NJ, USA) is taken into the peritoneal cavity through a stab incision at the lower end of the diastasis. The needle is pulled inside by a needle holder and assisting grasper. Then the intracorporeal suturing is started (Fig. 9.5). When the suturing is completed, both edges have been approximated and a new linea alba constructed (Fig. 9.6, 9.7, and 9.8).

Then the 10-mm trocar is replaced by a 12-mm optical trocar, and the whole surgical team changes their gloves. An appropriate size of tissue-separating mesh is chosen. Prolene 2–0 sutures (Ethicon; Somerville, NJ, USA) are taken with long threads left on the upper, middle, and lower parts of the mesh in the midline, using all aseptic measures. Then the mesh is rolled like a cigarette, held with the needle holder, and taken into the abdominal cavity through the 12-mm optical trocar.

The mesh is unrolled and the pre-tied Prolene sutures are taken out transfascially with a suture passer in the midline; this technique reduces the chance of neural entrapment and postoperative pain. Then intracorporeal transfascial suture fixation of the mesh is performed with Prolene 2–0 (Figs. 9.9, 9.10, and 9.11). It can also be done with PDS 2–0 to secure the position of the mesh as an intraperitoneal onlay mesh (IPOM).

Figure 9.12 shows postoperative images.

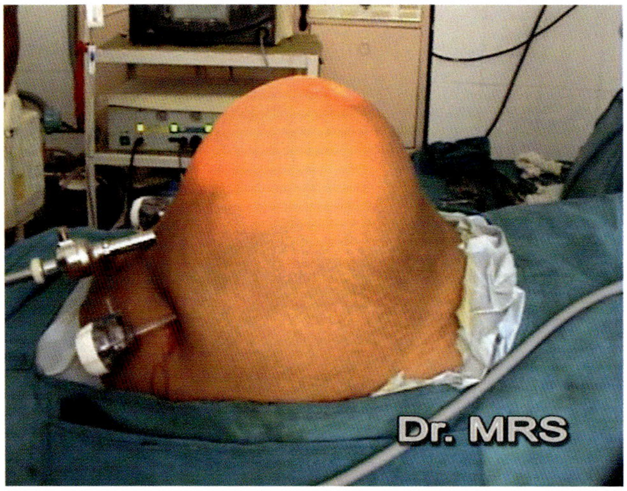

Fig. 9.1 Pneumoperitoneum

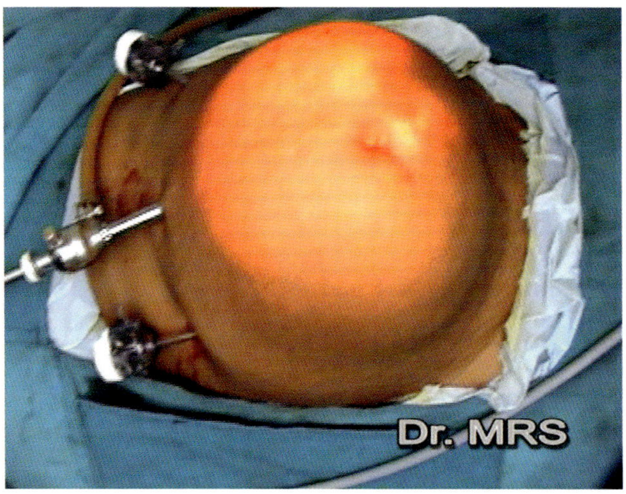

Fig. 9.2 Pneumoperitoneum done with a Veress needle. Three ports (one midline 10-mm port and two pararectal 5-mm ports) are inserted in the suprapubic region. The telescope is introduced into the 10-mm port

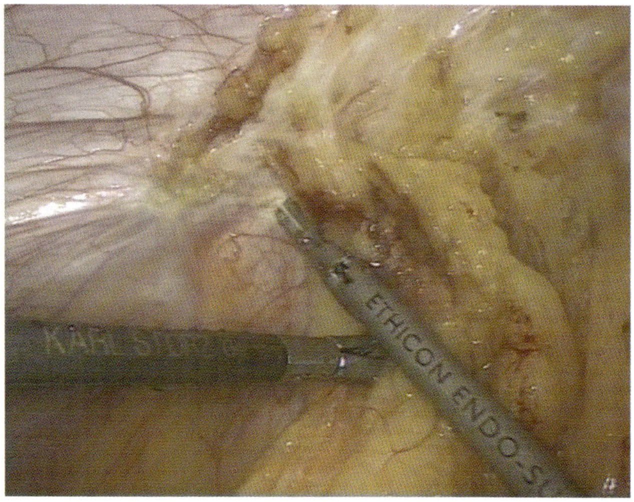

Fig. 9.3 Diagnostic laparoscopy and adhesiolysis

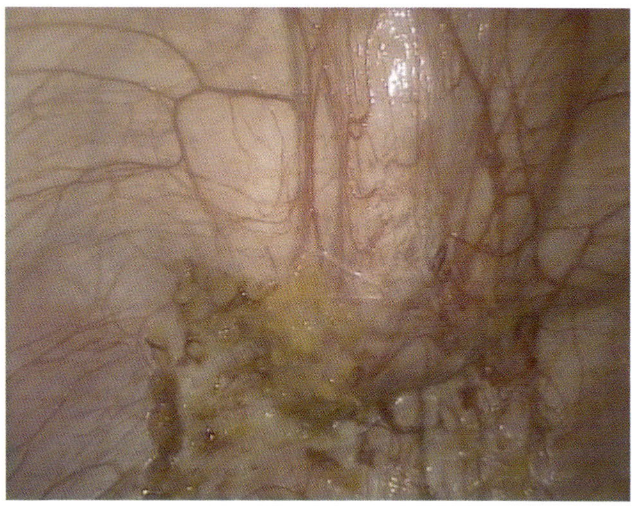

Fig. 9.4 The defect is made prominent by compression from outside

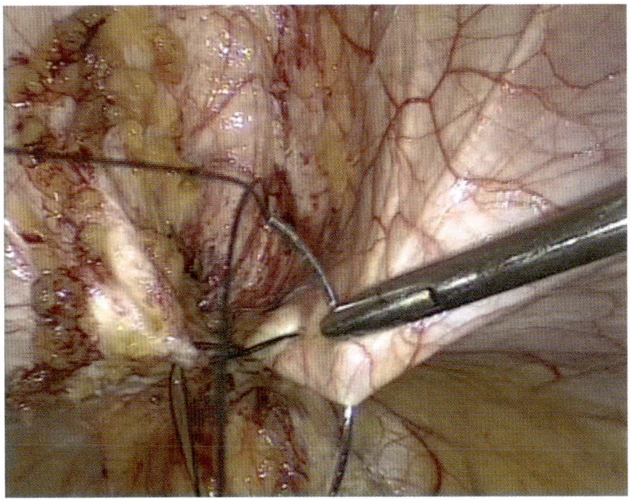

Fig. 9.5 Suturing of the edges of the defect is started with double loop 1 (4 metric) 48 mm ½ circle heavy round bodied Ethilon (monofilament polyamide black), creating a new linea alba

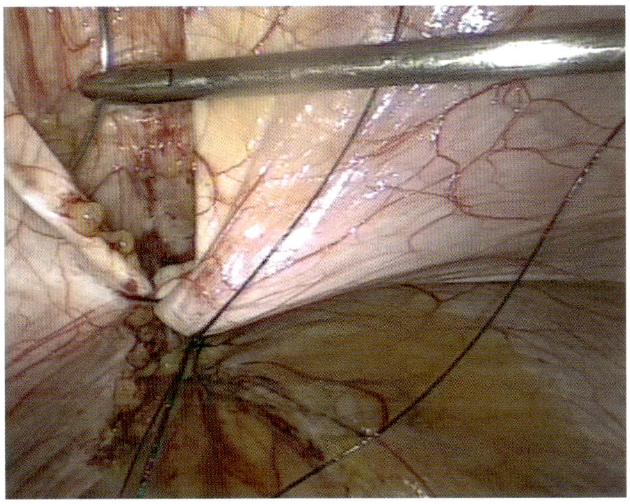

Fig. 9.6 Suturing in progress

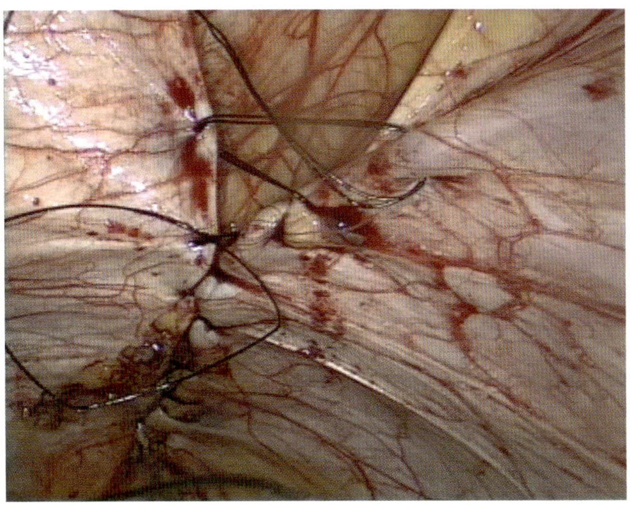

Fig. 9.7 Suturing near completion

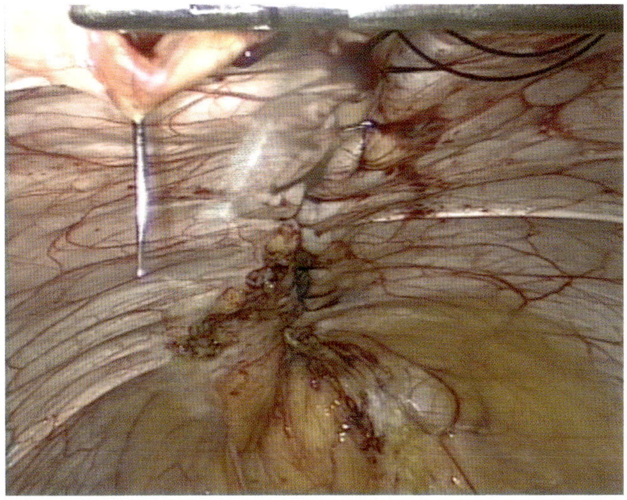

Fig. 9.8 Suturing completed

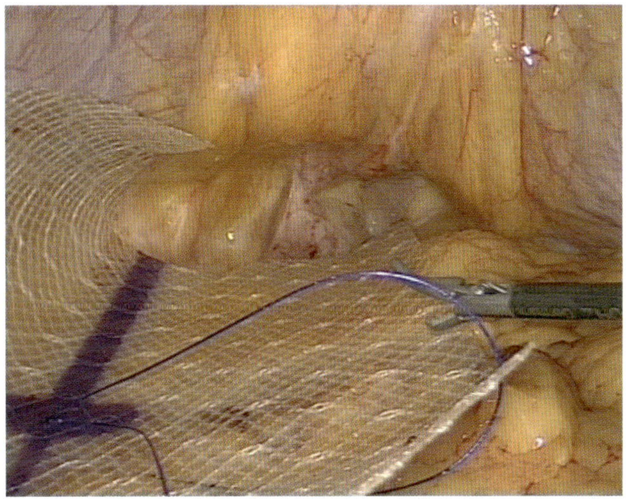

Fig. 9.9 Tissue-separating mesh is prepared for placement as intraperitoneal onlay mesh (IPOM)

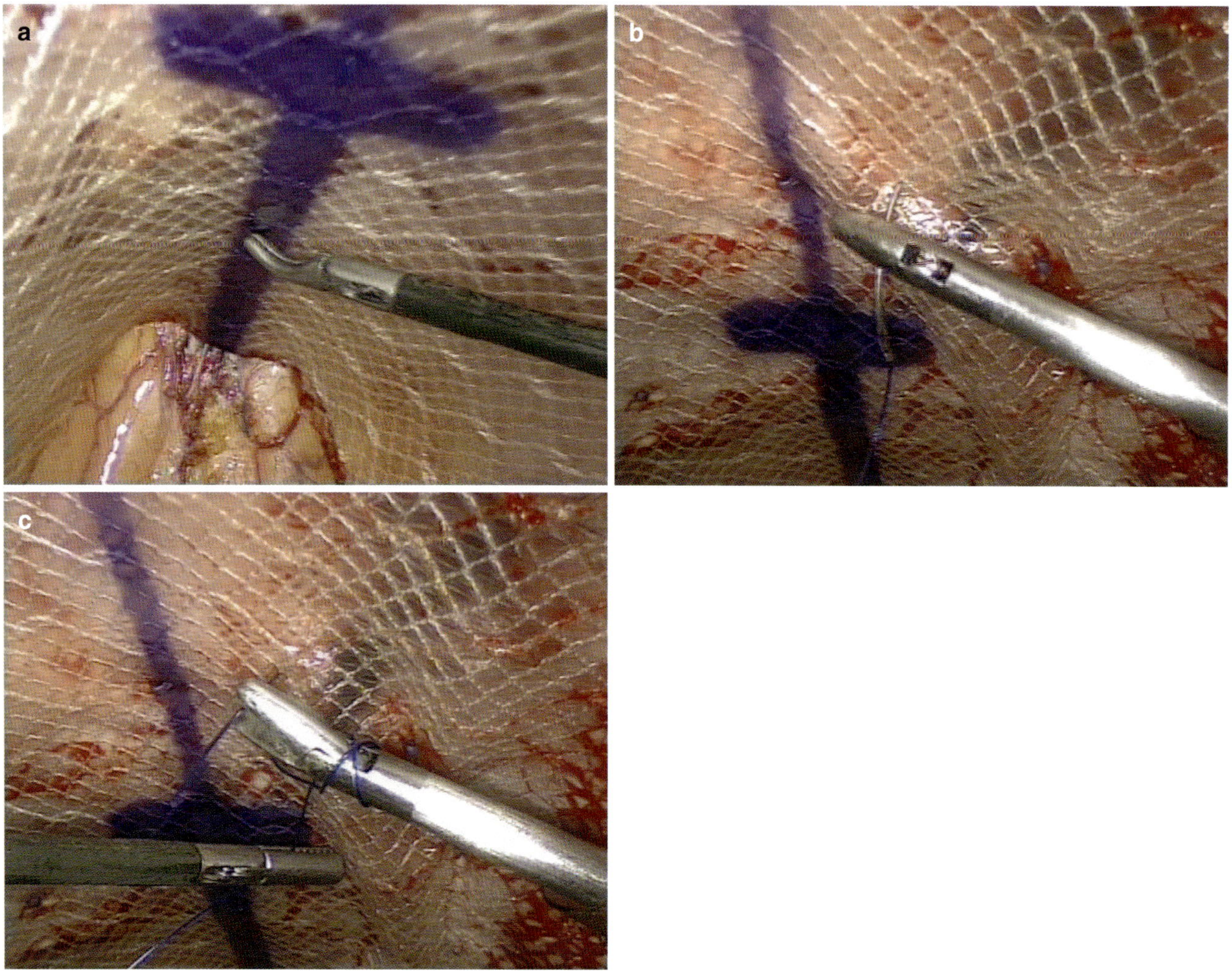

Fig. 9.10 (**a**–**c**) Mesh is fixed to the fascia tranversalis with intracorporeal transfascial suturing using 2–0 Prolene

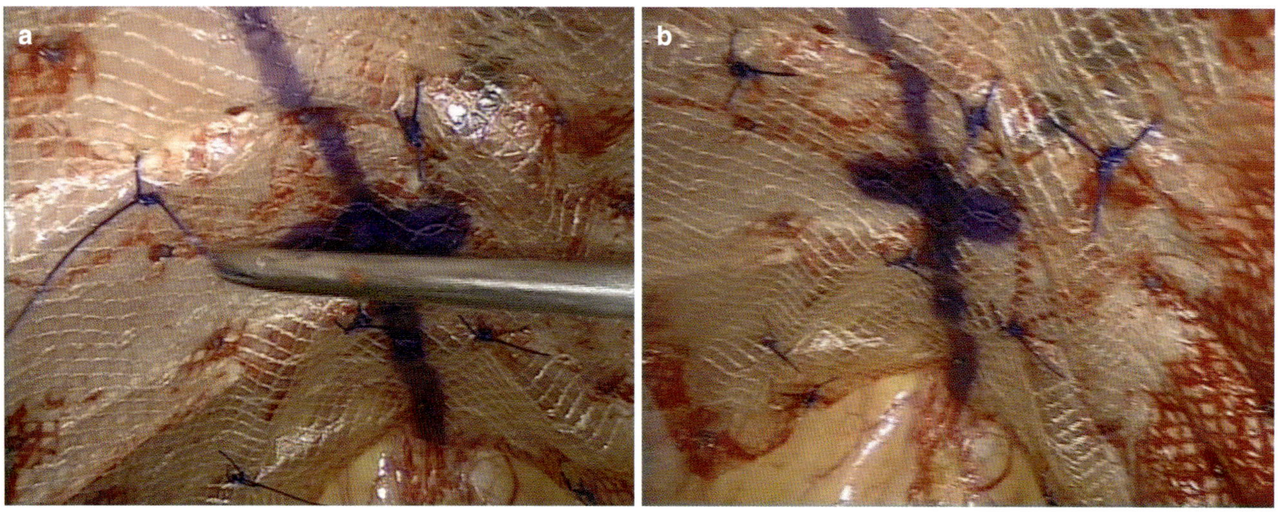

Fig. 9.11 (**a**, **b**) Completion of intracorporeal transfascial suturing

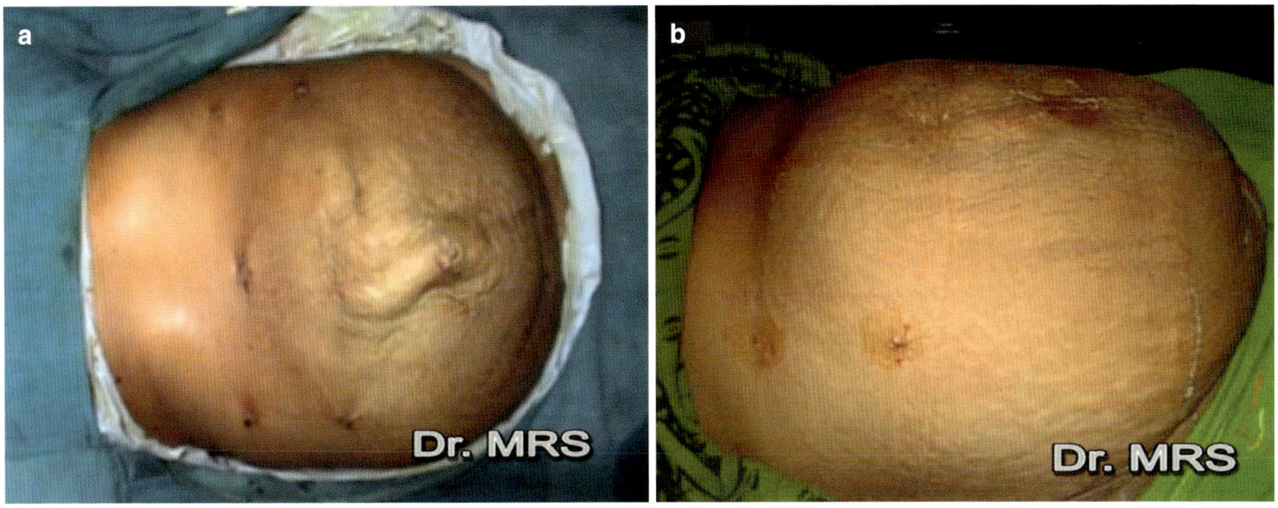

Fig. 9.12 (a, b) Immediate postoperative images of the external abdominal wall

Conclusions

The advent of endoscopy has yielded many novel procedures in all the specialties of surgery, but reports on the laparoscopic repair of diastasis recti are still very rare. Open procedures for diastasis recti have many complications such as hematoma, seroma formation, flap necrosis, hypertrophic scars, increased infection rate, and contour abnormalities that may be permanent. Laparoscopic repair, which is cosmetically more acceptable and lacks significant associated morbidities, is a promising future technique for the repair of diastasis recti.

References

1. Matei OA, Runkel N. A novel technique of midline mesh repair for umbilical hernia associated with diastasis recti. Surg Technol Int. 2014;24:183–7.
2. Veríssimo P, Nahas FX, Barbosa MV, de Carvalho Gomes HF, Ferreira LM. Is it possible to repair diastasis recti and shorten the aponeurosis at the same time? Aesthetic Plast Surg. 2014;38:379–86.
3. Akram J, Matzen SH. Rectus abdominis diastasis. J Plast Surg Hand Surg. 2014;48:163–9.
4. Tadiparthi S, Shokrollahi K, Doyle GS, Fahmy FS. Rectus sheath plication in abdominoplasty: assessment of its longevity and a review of the literature. J Plast Reconstr Aesthet Surg. 2012;65: 328–32.
5. Siddiky AH, Kapadia CR. Laparoscopic plication of the linea alba as a repair for diastasis recti – a mesh free approach. J Surg Case Rep. 2010;2010(5):3.
6. Brauman D. Diastasis recti: clinical anatomy. Plast Reconstr Surg. 2008;122:1564–9.
7. Core GB, Mizgala CL, Bowen 3rd JC, Vasconez LO. Endoscopic abdominoplasty with repair of diastasis recti and abdominal wall hernia. Clin Plast Surg. 1995;22:707–22.
8. Hughes KC, Weider L, Fischer J, Hopkins J, Antonetti A, Manders EK, Dunn E. Ventral hernia repair with simultaneous panniculectomy. Am Surg. 1996;62:678–81.
9. Asaadi M, Haramis HT. A simple technique for repair of rectus sheath defects. Ann Plast Surg. 1994;32:107–9.
10. Ranney B. Diastasis recti and umbilical hernia causes, recognition and repair. S D J Med. 1990;43(10):5–8.
11. Grinberg S. Repair of incisional midline hernia and diastasis of recti muscles. J Int Coll Surg. 1965;43:488–92.
12. Palanivelu C, Rangarajan M, Jategaonkar PA, Amar V, Gokul KS, Srikanth B. Laparoscopic repair of diastasis recti using the 'Venetian blinds' technique of plication with prosthetic reinforcement: a retrospective study. Hernia. 2009;13:287–92.
13. Journal of Women's Health Physical Therapy. Spring 2005;29(1): 11–16.

Endoscopic Cubital Tunnel Release

10

Nicholas M. Caggiano and Kristofer S. Matullo

Cubital tunnel syndrome (CuTS) is the second most common compressive neuropathy in the upper extremity, surpassed only by carpal tunnel syndrome. First described by Feindel and Stratford in 1958 [1], cubital tunnel syndrome is more common in women than in men and has an incidence of between 19 and 25 per 100,000 person-years [2]. Although the term "cubital tunnel syndrome" is commonly used to describe compression of the ulnar nerve at the elbow, it specifically refers to compression of the nerve within the cubital tunnel, more specifically by Osborne's ligament. Most patients can be treated with nonoperative modalities, including night splints, nerve glides, and activity modification by avoiding significant elbow flexion [3, 4]. Patients who are refractory to conservative therapy may require operative intervention. Surgical management includes in situ release; transposition performed subcutaneously, submuscularly, or intramuscularly; or medial epicondylectomy. More recently, endoscopic release of the cubital tunnel has become a popular choice among surgeons. Modern randomized, controlled trials have demonstrated equivalence among these methods of ulnar nerve decompression. Evidence has shown, however, that patients with a higher degree of preoperative neurologic compromise have worse outcomes [5].

N.M. Caggiano, MD
Department of Orthopaedic Surgery,
St. Luke's University Hospital,
801 Ostrum Street PPHP-2, Bethlehem, PA 18015, USA
e-mail: caggiano@slhn.org

K.S. Matullo, MD (✉)
Department of Orthopaedic Surgery,
St. Luke's University Hospital and Health Network,
801 Ostrum Street, PPH-2, Bethlehem, PA 18015, USA
e-mail: Kristofer.Matullo@sluhn.org

10.1 Anatomy

The ulnar nerve arises from the medial cord of the brachial plexus, receiving major contributions from the C8 and T1 spinal nerves, with a minor contribution from the C7 spinal nerve. The ulnar nerve exits the thoracic outlet medial to the axillary artery and is typically located between the axillary artery and axillary vein. It courses in the anterior compartment of the brachium between the brachialis and the medial head of the triceps, travelling medial to the brachial artery. A thick, fibrous band of tissue formed by the convergence of the medial intermuscular septum and the internal brachial ligament exists 8–9 cm proximal to the medial epicondyle of the humerus; it is often referred to as the arcade of Struthers. The ulnar nerve passes posterior to this arcade, transitioning from the anterior to the posterior compartment of the arm. The ulnar nerve does not provide any sensory or motor branches in the upper arm.

As the ulnar nerve approaches the elbow, it may course deep to an anomalous muscle, the anconeus epitrochlearis, if present. This muscle originates on the medial border of the olecranon and inserts on the medial epicondyle. The anconeus epitrochlearis is present in 34 % of the population, making it the most common anomalous muscle in the upper extremity [6]. The ulnar nerve then passes through the cubital tunnel, which is formed by the medial epicondyle, the olecranon process, the ulnar collateral ligament of the elbow, and the aponeurosis of the humeral and ulnar heads of the flexor carpi ulnaris (FCU). The two heads of the FCU are joined by an arch of fibrous tissue that runs from the medial epicondyle to the olecranon, referred to as the ligament of Osborne. Inside the cubital tunnel, the nerve supplies an average of one or two sensory branches to the elbow capsule [7].

The ulnar nerve then enters the anterior compartment of the forearm, passing under the aponeurosis of the FCU. It is at this point that motor innervation is supplied to the FCU and the medial half of the flexor digitorum profundus. In the forearm, most of the nerve's course is between the FCU and

E. Raposio (ed.), *Atlas of Endoscopic Plastic Surgery*, DOI 10.1007/978-3-319-19461-5_10

the flexor digitorum profundus. It provides no further innervation within the forearm.

The dorsal cutaneous branch of the ulnar nerve arises 5–10 cm proximal to the wrist flexion crease. It passes from the anterior compartment of the forearm to the dorsum of the hand at the ulnar styloid and supplies sensation to the ulnar-dorsal aspect of the hand and to the dorsal proximal and middle phalanges of the ring and small fingers.

The palmar cutaneous branch of the ulnar nerve has variable origin in the forearm, typically located distal to the dorsal cutaneous branch takeoff and proximal to the wrist flexion crease. It travels superficial to the transverse carpal ligament on the ulnar side of the ring finger metacarpal. The palmar cutaneous branch supplies sensation to the ulnar aspect of the palm.

The ulnar nerve proper enters the hand with the ulnar artery at Guyon's canal, which is bounded by the transverse carpal ligament, the volar carpal ligament, the pisiform, and the hamate. The ulnar nerve then divides into its superficial and deep terminal branches. The superficial branch innervates the palmaris brevis, as well as palmar sensation to the small finger and the ulnar aspect of the ring finger. The deep branch of the ulnar nerve innervates the hypothenar muscles, the third and fourth lumbricals, and the palmar and dorsal interossei. It also provides variable innervation to the deep head of the flexor pollicis brevis.

10.2 Etiology of Cubital Tunnel Syndrome

Ulnar neuropathy at the cubital tunnel is caused by compression of the nerve at the elbow. As the elbow moves from extension into flexion, Osborne's ligament stretches, causing a flattening and narrowing of the cubital tunnel [8]. The ulnar nerve also elongates as the elbow moves from 15° to 90°, and is relatively constant in length from 90° to 130° [9]. The combination of stretching of the ulnar nerve and narrowing of the cubital tunnel leads to compression of the ulnar nerve fibers. Compression decreases intraneural circulation, which in turn leads to paresthesias. As degeneration of the nerve becomes chronic, denervation of the muscles innervated by the ulnar nerve begins.

Patients with a history of trauma to the elbow may have altered anatomy that predisposes them to cubital tunnel syndrome. Malunion of the olecranon or distal humerus can decrease the volume of the tunnel available for safe passage of the nerve. Osteophytes from posttraumatic arthritis also can impinge on the nerve. Throwing athletes subject their elbows to valgus extension overload, which has been shown to cause osteophytes on the posteromedial olecranon [10].

10.3 History

Patients with cubital tunnel syndrome typically complain of tingling and numbness in the small finger and the ulnar half of the ring finger, both dorsally and volarly. These symptoms generally present sporadically and tend to increase in frequency as the compression continues. Complaints of tenderness at the medial aspect of the elbow are not uncommon. Patients may also complain of loss of grip strength or dexterity. Patients should be asked about difficulty with fine motor activities, such as buttoning a shirt or picking up coins off of a countertop. Weakness, fatigue, and loss of dexterity are secondary to denervation of the intrinsic muscles of the hand and are typically symptoms of more advanced disease. Wasting of the hypothenar musculature, intrinsics, and first dorsal interosseous muscle occurs in the later stages of disease progression.

The patient should be queried about positions of the affected upper extremity that exacerbate or alleviate the symptoms. Paresthesias with wrist flexion points to compression at Guyon's canal, whereas increased symptoms with overhead activities may suggest thoracic outlet syndrome. Numbness and tingling with elbow flexion implies compression at the cubital tunnel. Complaints of a painful popping sensation at the medial elbow with flexion may indicate that the ulnar nerve is subluxing over the medial epicondyle or the medial triceps is subluxing over the ulnar nerve.

Past medical history and social history should be elicited. Certain metabolic conditions such as hypothyroidism, diabetes mellitus, and vitamin deficiencies can manifest with similar symptoms. The patient's history should also be examined for trauma to the affected elbow, such as a supracondylar humerus fracture, which may lead to a tardy ulnar nerve palsy. Overhead throwing athletes may have ulnar nerve symptoms as a result of posteromedial olecranon osteophyte formation secondary to valgus extension overload.

10.4 Physical Examination

The diagnosis of cubital tunnel syndrome depends on a good and thorough physical examination. Visual inspection of the hand on the affected arm can yield important information. Chronic denervation of the intrinsic musculature can lead to clawing of the fingers, specifically the small and ring fingers. Wartenberg's sign, or abduction of the small finger, is caused by loss of innervation to the fourth palmar interosseous muscle and subsequent unopposed extension by the extensor digiti quinti. A Masse sign, flattening of the dorsal metacarpal arch over the small and ring fingers, is caused by weakness of the opponens digiti quinti secondary to denervation.

Provocative tests are designed to recreate the patient's subjective tingling and numbness. A Tinel's sign should be directly over the cubital tunnel in order to be considered positive. This test lacks specificity, but it has been shown to have the highest negative predictive value of all provocative tests at the cubital tunnel [11]. The elbow flexion test is performed by placing the patient's elbow in maximum flexion and supination for up to 60 s. A positive test is defined as re-creation of the patient's symptoms in the ulnar nerve distribution. The pressure provocation test is performed by placing the patient's elbow in 20° of flexion. The examiner places one or two fingers directly over the ulnar nerve at the cubital tunnel and applies pressure for 60 s. A positive result is similarly defined as recreation of the patient's symptoms in the ulnar nerve distribution. Both of these provocative tests have been widely used, but they are not highly sensitive [11] or particularly specific [12].

The scratch-collapse test has an accuracy rate of 98 % for compression of the ulnar nerve at the elbow [11]. The test is performed with the elbow in 90° of flexion and the arm adducted by the patient's side. The examiner tests the patient's ability to externally rotate against resistance at the shoulder. After a baseline assessment of strength is noted, the examiner gently scratches the skin over the cubital tunnel and subsequently reexamines the patient's ability to resist internal rotation. A positive result is defined by significant loss of external rotation strength compared with the baseline test.

Weakness of the intrinsic musculature of the hand can be elicited by having the patient perform a key pinch maneuver, holding a piece of paper between the thumb and index finger. The patient is instructed to hold the paper using only adduction of the thumb as the examiner attempts to pull the paper longitudinally out the patient's grasp. Patients with weakness of the adductor pollicis will compensate for their inability to adduct the thumb by flexing the interphalangeal joint via the flexor pollicis longus. This is known as the Froment's sign. Patients may exhibit hyperextension at the metatarsophalangeal joint, referred to as Jeanne's sign, as they recruit the extensor pollicis brevis to compensate for loss of thumb interphalangeal joint extension.

The McGowan scale can be used to grade ulnar nerve compression and provide patients with a likely prognosis following surgical intervention [13]. Grade I is defined as purely subjective complaints of tingling and numbness in the ulnar nerve distribution. Grade II includes sensory loss and intrinsic hand weakness. The worst prognosis for recovery occurs with McGowan Grade III, defined as muscle atrophy, severe sensory loss, and clawing of the fingers.

The Dellon classification groups patients into mild, moderate, or severe categories based on paresthesias and motor weakness [14]. Grade I patients have intermittent paresthesias and subjective weakness; they may have a positive Tinel's sign or elbow flexion test. Grade II patients also have periodic paresthesias but also have measurable weakness and a positive Tinel's sign and elbow flexion test. Grade III patients have persistent paresthesias, muscle atrophy, and abnormal muscle strength.

10.5 Diagnostic Studies

X-rays of the affected elbow should be obtained to uncover osseous pathology that may cause ulnar nerve compression. A cubitus valgus deformity may lead to a tardy ulnar nerve palsy due to prolonged tension and stretch on the nerve. Osteophytes from posttraumatic or degenerative arthritis can impinge on the ulnar nerve at the cubital tunnel. Ultrasound is a useful adjunct when there is suspicion that a soft-tissue mass may be the cause of compressive neuropathy. It is minimally invasive, relatively inexpensive, and also can provide dynamic evaluation of a subluxating nerve. MRI is rarely useful in the diagnosis of cubital tunnel syndrome.

Nerve conduction studies (NCS) provide useful confirmatory information in the setting of clinical diagnosis of cubital tunnel syndrome. NCS also can localize the cause of ulnar nerve compression in up to 96 % of cases [15]. Motor conduction velocities have been shown to be more sensitive than sensory studies [16]. Motor velocities less than 50 m per second from above the elbow to below the elbow are indicative of ulnar neuropathy at the elbow; velocities that are 10 m per second slower than in isolated segments above or below the elbow are also suggestive of ulnar neuropathy at the elbow. Controversy exists regarding the optimal position of the elbow during electrodiagnostic testing, however [17, 18].

10.6 Treatment

Conservative management is attempted primarily for all but the most severe cases. Night splints are designed to prevent elbow flexion while the patient is sleeping. Splints must be worn continuously at night for at least 6 months for long-lasting results [4]. Anti-inflammatory medications are used to decrease inflammation, with activity modification to decrease provocative positioning. Up to 89 % of patients with mild to moderate symptoms of cubital tunnel syndrome may recover with nonoperative treatment [19]. Contraindications for a trial of conservative treatment include evidence of chronic denervation on electrodiagnostic studies and overt muscle wasting; in these situations, operative intervention is warranted to preserve any remaining muscle function in the hand.

Operative treatment of cubital tunnel syndrome is based on decompression of the ulnar nerve. For patients without subluxation of the nerve, this can be performed as an in situ release of Osborne's ligament. This procedure is simple and reproducible; it minimizes trauma to the nerve and its vascular supply. Patients best suited for this procedure have activity-related symptoms without subluxation of the nerve.

In situ release via an endoscopic approach has become an acceptable alternative to open in situ release, allowing for a smaller incision and faster recovery [20]. Cadaveric studies have shown that the medial antebrachial nerve and the ulnar nerve branch to the FCU are both at risk during "open" release, but this risk may be mitigated by an endoscopic technique. Patient satisfaction following endoscopic cubital tunnel release is at least equivalent to open in situ release [21, 22], and patients reported relief of pain and paresthesias sooner in the postoperative period [23]. Evidence has also shown earlier return to work with endoscopic release than with anterior transposition [22].

Patients with subluxation of the ulnar nerve over the medial epicondyle typically are not candidates for simple in situ decompression, as decompression does not address—and may increase—subluxation. Options for these patients include subcutaneous, intramuscular, or submuscular transposition. Transposition places the ulnar nerve anterior to the axis of elbow flexion, effectively increasing its relative length and decreasing the tension on it. This procedure is also indicated when space-occupying lesions such as osteophytes or soft-tissue masses are located within the cubital tunnel. Typically patients undergoing revision cubital tunnel release are also treated with ulnar nerve transposition. The choice between subcutaneous versus submuscular transposition is mostly one of surgeon preference. Randomized controlled trials and meta-analysis reviews have failed to show conclusive evidence in support of either subcutaneous or submuscular transposition [5, 24–28].

Medial epicondylectomy is an alternative to in situ decompression or anterior transposition. Advocates of this procedure state that it removes the bony compressive elements at the cubital tunnel and relieves the tensile stress on the ulnar nerve [29] without extensive dissection of the nerve and potential compromise of its vascularity [30]. There have been reports of pain and instability following medial epicondylectomy [31, 32], newer techniques such as partial or oblique epicondylectomy have shown promising outcomes [33, 34].

10.7 Complications

Complications following surgical treatment for cubital tunnel syndrome include incomplete release, instability, pain, postoperative scar formation, and iatrogenic nerve injury [28, 33, 35]. Risk factors for revision surgery include age greater than 50 years, submuscular transposition, symptoms lasting longer than 6 months, and electrodiagnostic evidence of denervation prior to surgical intervention [5, 35, 36]. Patients with worse preoperative symptoms must be counseled before the intervention to expect less than optimal results [22].

10.8 Surgical Technique

The procedure described below for endoscopic cubital tunnel release is an adaptation from the surgical description originally published by Cobb [20].

10.8.1 Anesthesia and Positioning

Typically, the procedure is performed under general anesthesia in an operating room suite. The patient is placed supine on a general operating room table and a hand table is utilized (Fig. 10.1).

10.8.2 Landmarks

Figure 10.2 illustrates typical preoperative marking of the arm.

10.8.3 Procedure

The skin incision is made with a #15 blade and continued, raising full-thickness anterior and posterior flaps toward the medial epicondyle. Care is taken to identify crossing venous structures; hemostasis is maintained with electrocautery. A branch of the medial antebrachial cutaneous nerve may be identified, but it is not typically encountered.

Figures 10.3, 10.4, 10.5, 10.6, 10.7, 10.8, 10.9, 10.10, 10.11, and 10.12 illustrate the rest of the procedure.

At the end of the procedure, the tourniquet is deflated and hemostasis is obtained under direct visualization with pressure and electrocautery. The wounds are copiously irrigated with a normal saline solution and closed in a layered fashion. The area is injected with local anesthetic (such as 1 % lidocaine with 1:100,000 epinephrine) for postoperative pain control. The wounds are covered with a nonadherent gauze, sterile gauze, and a compressive overwrap.

10.8.4 Postoperative Care

The patient is given a prescription for pain medication as required. Nonsteroidal anti-inflammatory medications are typically avoided for the first 48–72 h to minimize postoperative hematoma formation. The patient is instructed to elevate the hand and elbow and apply ice for 30 min every 2 h for the first 24 h, except while sleeping. The patient may remove the dressings on postoperative day 2 and shower normally, patting the elbow dry, but the elbow should not be soaked in standing water such as a bathtub or swimming pool while the sutures are in place. Light activity is allowed when comfortable, but heavy activity should be avoided. The sutures are removed 10–14 days after surgery, when the incisions are healed. Activity is then progressed according to the tolerance of the patient.

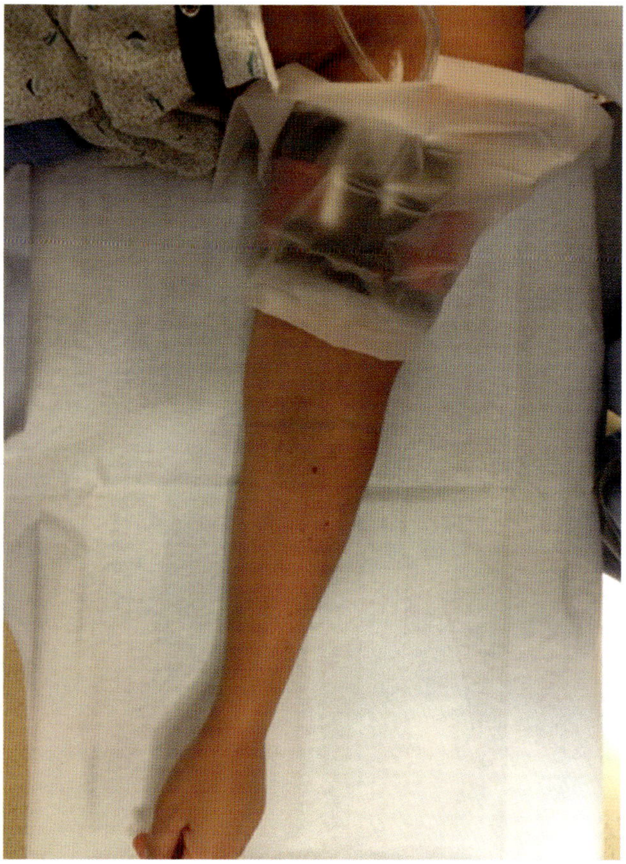

Fig. 10.1 A well-padded pneumatic tourniquet is placed on the upper arm and is typically inflated to 250 mmHg. The remainder of the arm is prepped and draped in standard fashion

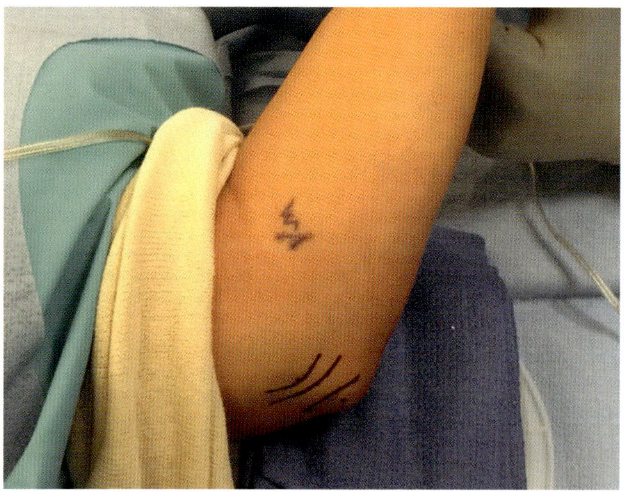

Fig. 10.2 The medial epicondyle of the arm is marked, as is the tip of the olecranon on the medial aspect. With the arm held in 45–60° of flexion, the usual course of the ulnar nerve is drawn; it can typically be palpated under the skin. If the ulnar nerve subluxes, the arm is held with the nerve in a reduced position, typically in 45° of flexion. The incision is drawn, extending from just proximal to the medial epicondyle to 2 cm distal. This incision is located slightly anterior to the course of the ulnar nerve

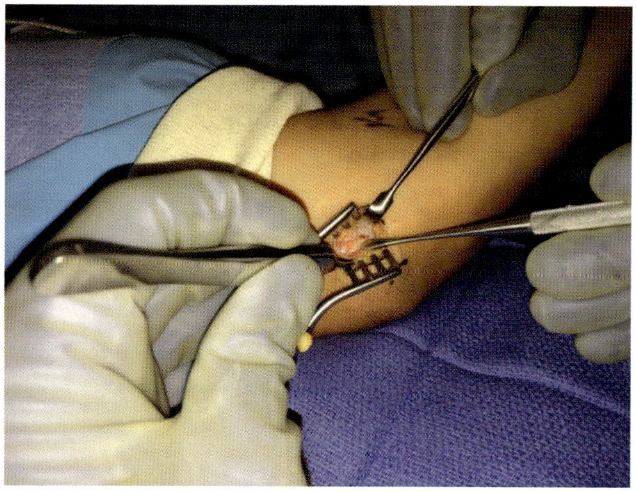

Fig. 10.3 The fascia overlying the flexor carpi ulnaris (FCU) muscle is identified at the distal extent of the incision and marks the depth of the dissection. The fascia of Osborne's ligament is divided over the cubital tunnel by removing it from the posterior aspect of the medial epicondyle until the ulnar nerve is identified

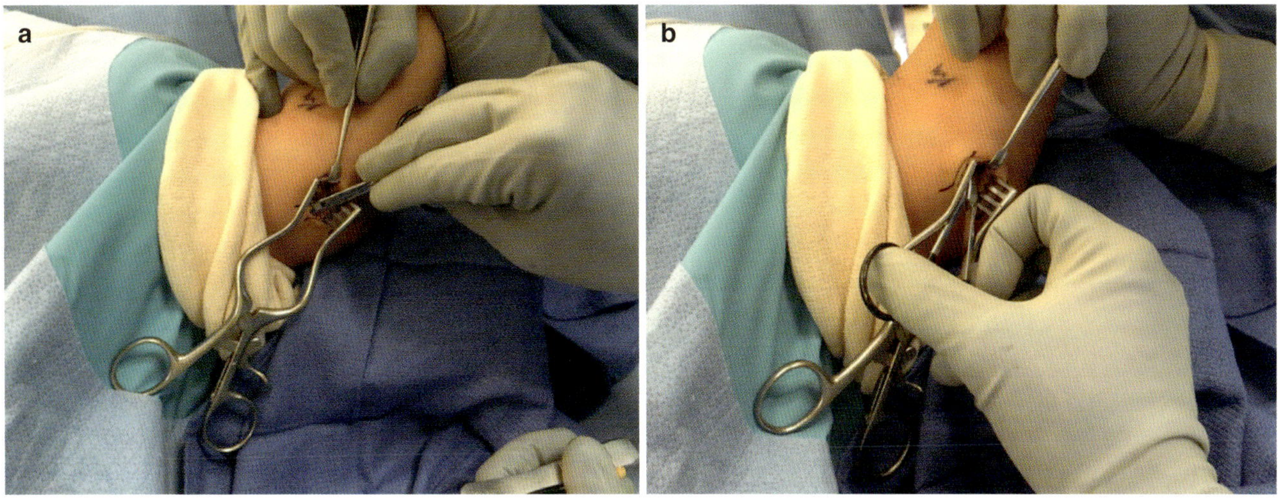

Fig. 10.4 (**a**, **b**) A blunt tenotomy scissors is used to develop a pocket superficial to the fascia and Osborne's ligament both proximally and distally. Any venous structures identified are either retracted or coagulated. Proximally, the ulnar nerve can often be visualized emerging from the arcade of Struthers; distally, it passes deep to the fascia of the FCU

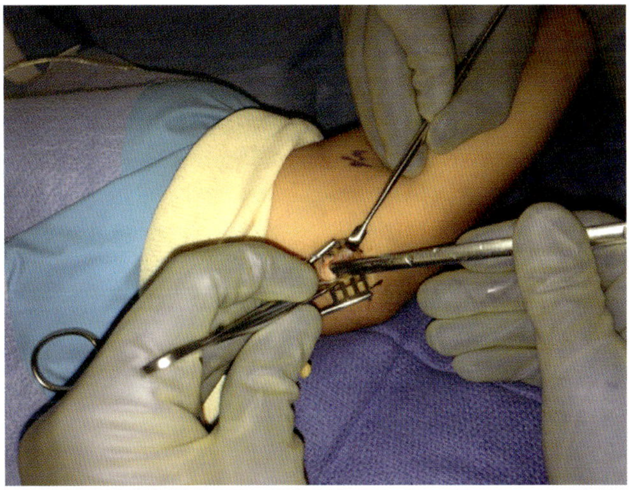

Fig. 10.5 Proximally, a blunt-tipped dissector is inserted deep to the fascia, creating a pocket for the trocar and camera

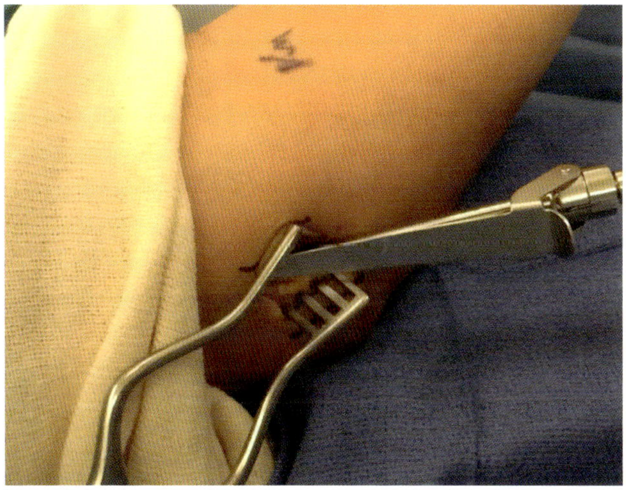

Fig. 10.6 The trocar is inserted deep to the fascia and superficial to the ulnar nerve. Slots within the posterior cannula should be aligned along the course of the ulnar nerve to ensure maximal nerve protection. The metal soft-tissue protection sleeve should be superficial to the fascia but deep to the subcutaneous tissues

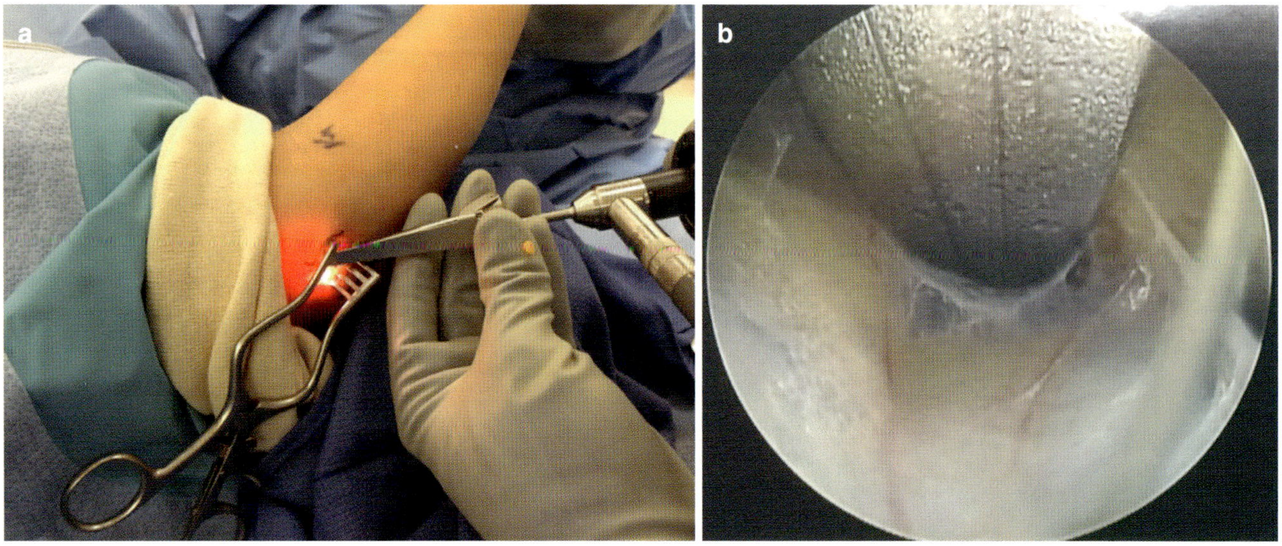

Fig. 10.7 (**a**, **b**) The camera is inserted between the fascia and the protection sleeve to verify that no aberrant nerve or vascular structures are present within the path of the intended nerve release. The camera is inserted into the trocar sleeve

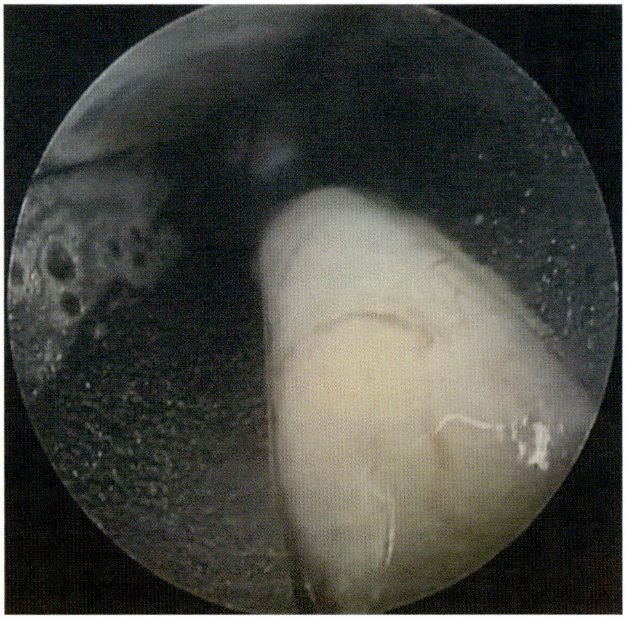

Fig. 10.8 The ulnar nerve is visualized through the posterior slots of the cannula, and the trocar is rotated to ensure that the ulnar nerve is safely protected along its entire course

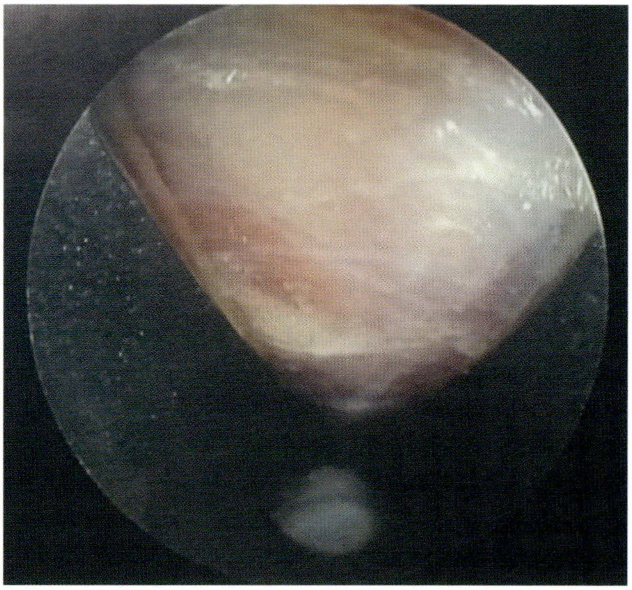

Fig. 10.9 The camera should be rotated to visualize the undersurface of the fascia, ensuring that nerve or vascular structures are not trapped between the trocar and the fascia

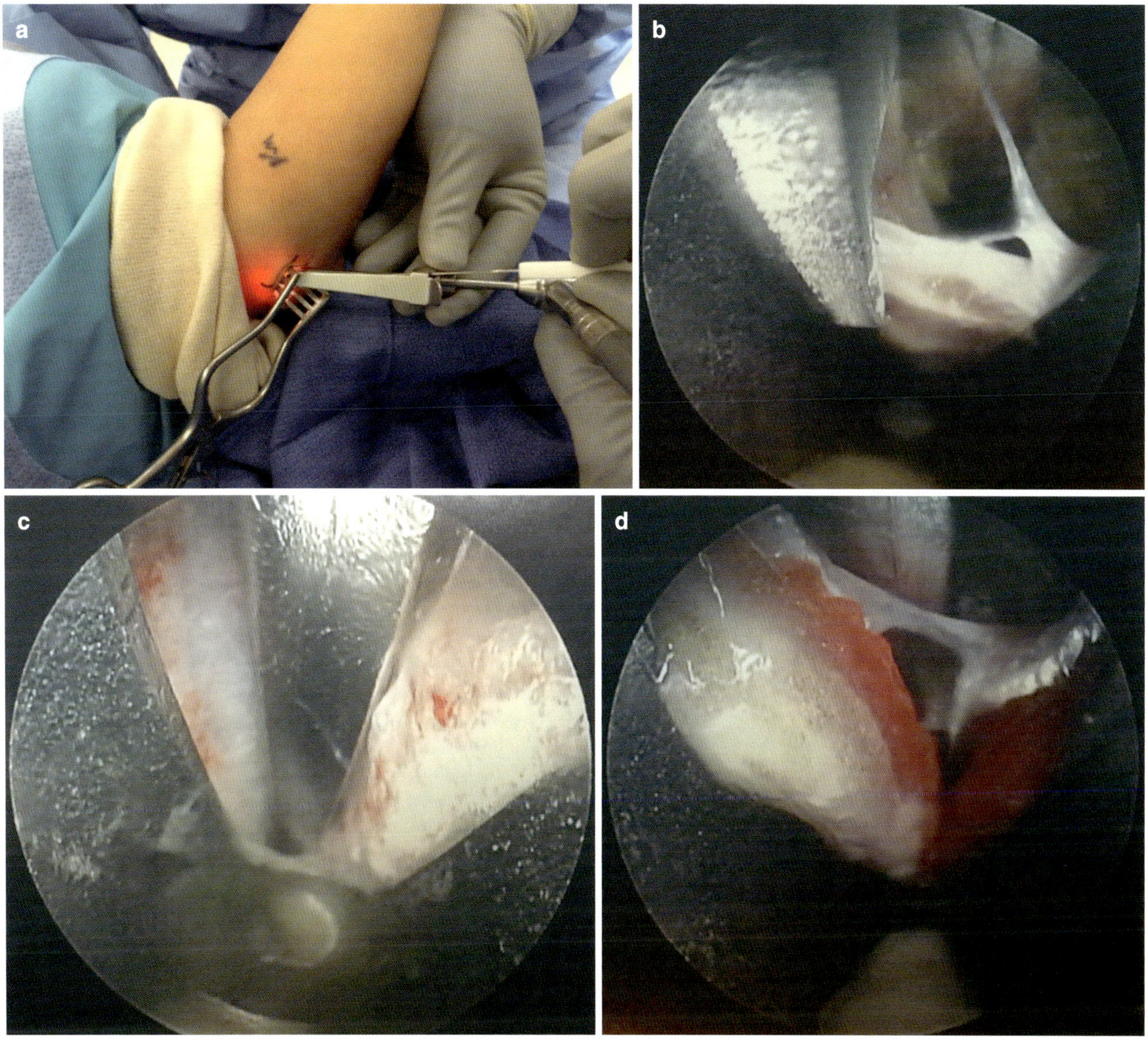

Fig. 10.10 (**a–d**) Under direct visualization, an antegrade cutting knife is inserted through the cutting slot and is used to divide the fascia. The knife, camera, and cannula are removed and the area is inspected to ensure that the fascia has been divided and no injury to the ulnar nerve has occurred

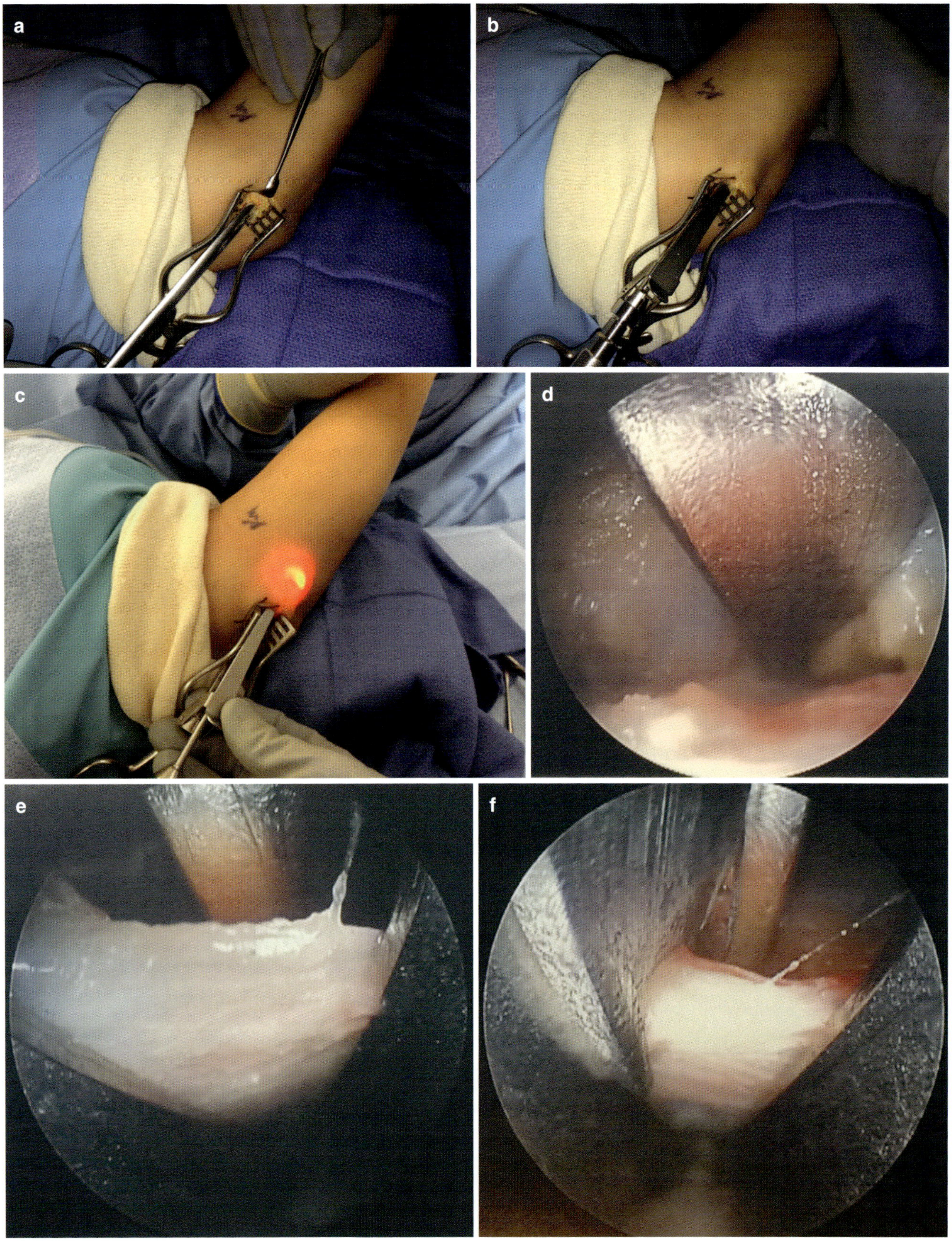

Fig. 10.11 (**a**–**f**) The procedure is replicated in the distal direction, ensuring that the ulnar nerve is released to the level of the motor branch to the FCU muscle

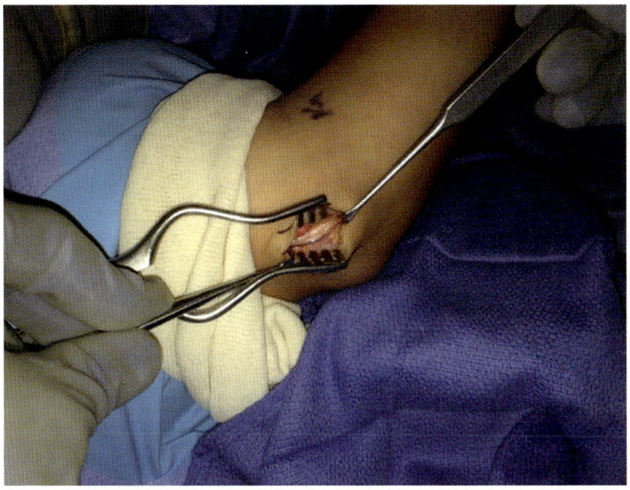

Fig. 10.12 After release proximally and distally, the elbow is brought through a full arc of motion from extension to flexion while the ulnar nerve is monitored for subluxation; if the ulnar nerve subluxes, transposition of the nerve should be considered

References

1. Feindel W, Stratford J. Cubital tunnel compression in tardy ulnar palsy. Can Med Assoc J. 1958;78:351–3.
2. Latinovic R, Gulliford MC, Hughes RA. Incidence of common compressive neuropathies in primary care. J Neurol Neurosurg Psychiatry. 2006;77:263–5.
3. Shah CM, Calfee RP, Gelberman RH, Goldfarb CA. Outcomes of rigid night splinting and activity modification in the treatment of cubital tunnel syndrome. J Hand Surg Am. 2013;38:1125–30.
4. Seror P. Treatment of ulnar nerve palsy at the elbow with a night splint. J Bone Joint Surg Br. 1993;75:322–7.
5. Charles YP, Coulet B, Rouzaud JC, Daures JP, Chammas M. Comparative clinical outcomes of submuscular and subcutaneous transposition of the ulnar nerve for cubital tunnel syndrome. J Hand Surg Am. 2009;34:866–74.
6. Masear VR, Hill Jr JJ, Cohen SM. Ulnar compression neuropathy secondary to the anconeus epitrochlearis muscle. J Hand Surg Am. 1988;13:720–4.
7. Bekler H, Riansuwan K, Vroemen JC, McKean J, Wolfe VM, Rosenwasser MP. Innervation of the elbow joint and surgical perspectives of denervation: a cadaveric anatomic study. J Hand Surg Am. 2008;33:740–5.
8. Apfelberg DB, Larson SJ. Dynamic anatomy of the ulnar nerve at the elbow. Plast Reconstr Surg. 1973;51:79–81.
9. James J, Sutton LG, Werner FW, Basu N, Allison MA, Palmer AK. Morphology of the cubital tunnel: an anatomical and biomechanical study with implications for treatment of ulnar nerve compression. J Hand Surg Am. 2011;36:1988–95.
10. Wilson FD, Andrews JR, Blackburn TA, McCluskey G. Valgus extension overload in the pitching elbow. Am J Sports Med. 1983;11:83–8.
11. Cheng CJ, Mackinnon-Patterson B, Beck JL, Mackinnon SE. Scratch collapse test for evaluation of carpal and cubital tunnel syndrome. J Hand Surg Am. 2008;33:1518–24.
12. Rayan GM, Jensen C, Duke J. Elbow flexion test in the normal population. J Hand Surg Am. 1992;17:86–9.
13. McGowan AJ. The results of transposition of the ulnar nerve for traumatic ulnar neuritis. J Bone Joint Surg Br. 1950;32:293–301.
14. Dellon AL. Review of treatment results for ulnar nerve entrapment at the elbow. J Hand Surg Am. 1989;14:688–700.
15. Lee DH, Claussen GC, Oh S. Clinical nerve conduction and needle electromyography studies. J Am Acad Orthop Surg. 2004;12:276–87.
16. Kothari MJ, Heistand M, Rutkove SB. Three ulnar nerve conduction studies in patients with ulnar neuropathy at the elbow. Arch Phys Med Rehabil. 1998;79:87–9.
17. Nelson RM. Effects of elbow position on motor conduction velocity of the ulnar nerve. Phys Ther. 1980;60:780–3.
18. Harding C, Halar E. Motor and sensory ulnar nerve conduction velocities: effect of elbow position. Arch Phys Med Rehabil. 1983;64:227–32.
19. Svernlov B, Larsson M, Rehn K, Adolfsson L. Conservative treatment of the cubital tunnel syndrome. J Hand Surg Eur. 2009;34:201–7.
20. Cobb TK. Endoscopic cubital tunnel release. J Hand Surg Am. 2010;35:1690–7.
21. Watts AC, Bain GI. Patient-rated outcome of ulnar nerve decompression: a comparison of endoscopic and open in situ decompression. J Hand Surg Am. 2009;34:1492–8.
22. Cobb TK, Walden AL, Merrell PT, Lemke JH. Setting expectations following endoscopic cubital tunnel release. Hand. 2014;9:356–63.
23. Hoffmann R, Siemionow M. The endoscopic management of cubital tunnel syndrome. J Hand Surg Am. 2006;31:23–9.
24. Zhong W, Zhang W, Zheng X, Li S, Shi J. Comparative study of different surgical transposition methods for ulnar nerve entrapment at the elbow. J Int Med Res. 2011;39:1766–72.
25. Zarezadeh A, Shemshaki H, Nourbakhsh M, Etemadifar MR, Moeini M, Mazoochian F. Comparison of anterior subcutaneous and submuscular transposition of ulnar nerve in treatment of cubital tunnel syndrome: a prospective randomized trial. J Res Med Sci. 2012;17:745–9.
26. Caliandro P, La Torre G, Padua R, Giannini F, Padua L. Treatment for ulnar neuropathy at the elbow. Cochrane Database Syst Rev. 2012;7, CD006839.
27. Macadam SA, Gandhi R, Bezuhly M, Lefaivre KA. Simple decompression versus anterior subcutaneous and submuscular transposition of the ulnar nerve for cubital tunnel syndrome: a meta-analysis. J Hand Surg Am. 2008;33:1314.
28. Nellans K, Tang P. Evaluation and treatment of failed ulnar nerve release at the elbow. Orthop Clin North Am. 2012;43:487–94.
29. Hicks D, Toby EB. Ulnar nerve strains at the elbow: the effect of in situ decompression and medial epicondylectomy. J Hand Surg Am. 2002;27:1026–31.
30. Heithoff SJ, Millender LH, Nalebuff EA, Petruska Jr AJ. Medial epicondylectomy for the treatment of ulnar nerve compression at the elbow. J Hand Surg Am. 1990;15:22–9.
31. Kaempffe FA, Farbach J. A modified surgical procedure for cubital tunnel syndrome: partial medial epicondylectomy. J Hand Surg Am. 1998;23:492–9.
32. Cole RJ, Jemison DM, Hayes CW. Anterior elbow dislocation following medial epicondylectomy: a case report. J Hand Surg Am. 1994;19:614–6.
33. Muermans S, De Smet L. Partial medial epicondylectomy for cubital tunnel syndrome: outcome and complications. J Shoulder Elbow Surg. 2002;11:248–52.
34. Osei DA, Padegimas EM, Calfee RP, Gelberman RH. Outcomes following modified oblique medial epicondylectomy for treatment of cubital tunnel syndrome. J Hand Surg Am. 2013;38:336–43.
35. Jackson LC, Hotchkiss RN. Cubital tunnel surgery. Complications and treatment of failures. Hand Clin. 1996;12:449–56.
36. Ehsan A, Hanel DP. Recurrent or persistent cubital tunnel syndrome. J Hand Surg Am. 2012;37:1910–2.

11 Endoscopic Carpal Tunnel Release

Daniel M. Avery III and Kristofer S. Matullo

Carpal tunnel syndrome (CTS) was first described by Sir James Paget in 1854 [1, 2]. Today, it is recognized as the most common upper extremity compressive neuropathy, occurring under the transverse carpal ligament of the wrist and causing median nerve symptoms. The compression can be idiopathic or can result from trauma or systemic illness [3–5]. Sir James Learmouth performed the first release of the transverse carpal ligament in 1933 for traumatic median nerve compression following a distal radius fracture [6].

11.1 Anatomy

The transverse carpal ligament is the distal thickened flexor retinaculum found in the wrist. The hook of the hamate and pisiform delineate its ulnar boundaries; the scaphoid tubercle with trapezial ridge delineates its radial boundary [5, 7]. The median nerve is the most palmar structure within the tunnel. Deep and radial is the flexor pollicis longus. On the ulnar side are the four flexor digitorum superficialis tendons, and the most dorsal contents are the four flexor digitorum profundus tendons.

11.2 History

Carpal tunnel syndrome is primarily a clinical diagnosis. Sensory changes in the median nerve distribution are the first effects to appear, causing numbness or tingling on the palmar aspect of the thumb, index finger, and long finger, with variable effects to the radial aspect of the ring finger. Occasionally, patients complain of a "sandpaper" sensation in the hand while manipulating objects. The sensory deficit or changes can range from mild feelings that occur only at night (causing the patient to wake up and feel a need to shake out the affected hand) to symptoms that occur constantly throughout the day, with exacerbation during use of the hand.

Pain and weakness are also common complaints of patients with CTS. Pain can be felt over the carpal tunnel, radiating into the hand towards the thenar eminence, or in more severe cases, radiating proximally up the arm. Weakness or difficulty with fine motor movements commonly occurs as the disease progresses. Patients will admit to dropping even light objects, or experiencing problems using keys or manipulating buttons or coins. Examining the thenar musculature can give an indication of the severity of the compression, as atrophy typically represents thenar muscle loss.

11.3 Etiology

CTS has many possible causes but is most commonly idiopathic. It affects between 1 and 10 % of the population and is more common in obese, older, inactive individuals [8]. Traumatic CTS can occur following a distal radius fracture with dorsal displacement of the distal segment, or with other less common injuries such as a perilunate dislocation. Reduction of the fracture may improve symptoms, but persistent swelling can continue after fracture healing, eventually requiring surgical intervention.

Systemic causes can include pregnancy, obesity, diabetes, hypothyroidism, amyloidosis, systemic lupus erythematosus, and rheumatoid arthritis [3–5, 8]. These processes often can be part of a multifactorial cause or can be a cause of transient symptoms. Space-occupying lesions such as infection or tumor can also contribute to median nerve compression [9].

D.M. Avery III, MD
Department of Orthopaedic Surgery, St. Luke's University Hospital, 801 Ostrum Street, PPH-2, Bethlehem, PA 18015, USA
e-mail: Daniel.Avery@sluhn.org

K.S. Matullo, MD (✉)
Department of Orthopaedic Surgery,
St. Luke's University Hospital and Health Network,
801 Ostrum Street, PPH-2, Bethlehem, PA 18015, USA
e-mail: Kristofer.Matullo@sluhn.org

E. Raposio (ed.), *Atlas of Endoscopic Plastic Surgery*, DOI 10.1007/978-3-319-19461-5_11

11.4 Physical Examination

A thorough physical examination of the hand, the neck, and the upper extremity is important for accurate diagnosis. Cervical radiculopathy commonly masquerades as CTS, but it also can be part of the "double crush" phenomenon of concomitant cervical and median nerve compression. Radicular symptoms moving proximal to distal, weakness in upper extremity musculature, and other positive physical examination maneuvers such as a Spurling's sign, Lhermitte's sign, or Hoffman's sign should shift the examiner's focus toward cervical spine pathology.

The hand may appear normal in patients with early or mild CTS. In advanced stages, with severe compression and axonal degeneration, marked atrophy of the thenar musculature may be present. This atrophy may be more difficult to appreciate when bilateral extremities are affected, and it may be confused with age-related changes.

Palpation of the thenar eminence may sometimes demonstrate an indentation from chronic muscle wasting. Commonly, there are no areas of tenderness, but occasional patients have pain over the carpal tunnel along the course of the median nerve. Atrophy of the first two lumbricals, those to the index and long finger, may also be noted. Atrophy of other muscles of the hand, such as the first dorsal interosseous, the dorsal and volar intrinsics, or the lumbricals to the ring and small finger, should also be evaluated to rule out other generalized neuropathies such as diabetic or ulnar neuropathy.

The strength of the opponens pollicis, abductor pollicis brevis, and flexor pollicis brevis should be assessed. Weakness of palmar abduction or opposition commonly reflects carpal tunnel compression. Because of the dual innervation of the flexor pollicis brevis through the recurrent branch of the median nerve and the ulnar nerve, however, strength can appear normal in this muscle even with advanced cases of CTS.

Provocative physical examination maneuvers for CTS include Tinel's sign, Phalen's test, and Durkan's compression test. Tinel's sign is evoked by percussion over the median nerve at the wrist, with a positive finding of sensory disturbance (usually tingling) in the median nerve distribution. Sensitivity ranges from 48 to 73 % and specificity ranges from 30 to 94 % [10–12]. Phalen's test requires the patient to hold both wrists in a volarly flexed position for up to 60 s. Paresthesias in the median nerve distribution are considered a positive test. Gellman et al. [13] supported this maneuver by showing that wrist flexion increased the pressure within the carpal tunnel by up to 3 times. The Durkan compression test manually recreates increased pressure within the carpal tunnel by having the clinician press directly over the carpal tunnel for up to 30 s, evaluating for paresthesias within the fingers. The sensitivity of the Durkan compression test has been reported to be 89 %, and specificity to be 96 %; it is considered by some to be a better provocative test than Tinel's sign or Phalen's test [14, 15].

11.5 Diagnostic Studies

Radiographs of the affected hand and wrist are not typically obtained in the initial office visit, but in the setting of recent or prior trauma or a history of inflammatory or significant degenerative arthritis, posteroanterior (PA), lateral, and carpal tunnel views may demonstrate fracture malunion or a space-occupying lesion. CT scans are not typically obtained. Ultrasound can be useful for evaluating the presence of a mass and has the advantage of demonstrating flexor tendon movement dynamically. MRI is generally used only for advanced imaging of a soft-tissue mass, if present.

Nerve conduction studies (NCS) and electromyography (EMG) are helpful in confirming CTS while simultaneously evaluating for more proximal sites of nerve entrapment or generalized pathology. Positive NCS findings for CTS include an increase in the distal motor and sensory latencies, decreased amplitude, and slower conduction velocities. The EMG may demonstrate increased insertional activity, positive sharp waves, fibrillations, and decreased motor recruitment as the disease progresses. The severity of CTS graded by EMG and NCS can help guide the physician and patient regarding expectations. With increasing severity of CTS, the recovery time may increase and the chance of complete resolution of subjective symptoms and objective findings decreases. There is a subset of patients (16–34 %) with clinical CTS but normal electrodiagnostic studies, however. For these patients, the clinical history and examination should determine the diagnosis and guide treatment [16–18].

11.6 Treatment

Symptom severity guides the treatment for CTS. In mild cases without thenar atrophy or acute compression, splinting the wrist in a neutral position during sleep is evaluated. The splints help reduce the pressure within the carpal tunnel due to abnormal wrist positioning and may eliminate symptoms. Corticosteroid injections into the carpal tunnel help to decrease the tenosynovitis, but typically provide only temporary relief for most patients. Injections may be used as a diagnostic tool in cases of concomitant cervical disease or recurrent carpal tunnel symptoms, however, as patients who describe significant relief after corticosteroid injections within the carpal tunnel typically have better results after surgical decompression [19].

Carpal tunnel release is indicated for patients with persistent symptoms, a presentation of severe compression, thenar atrophy, or denervation changes on electrodiagnostic studies. Currently, carpal tunnel release may be performed by open, mini-open, or endoscopic techniques. Despite the advances in endoscopy, many surgeons still favor open carpal tunnel release, and it is still the procedure of choice for recurrent CTS or patients with additional pathology, such as the presence of a mass. Endoscopic release has been shown to have excellent results, with less postoperative pain, scar tenderness, thumb weakness, and a quicker return to work [2]. All techniques typically result in high patient satisfaction, reduction in paresthesias, variable return of motor function, and a relatively low complication rate [2, 20].

11.7 Complications

Complications following endoscopic carpal tunnel release are relatively rare. They include incomplete release, ulnar nerve symptoms, painful scar, and recurrent tenosynovitis [20, 21]. For the Chow two-incision endoscopic technique (the basis for the technique presented in this chapter), reported rates of recurrence, incomplete release, and transient ulnar nerve symptoms are all less than 1 % [20].

11.8 Surgical Technique

11.8.1 Anesthesia

The endoscopic carpal tunnel release procedure historically has been performed under either general anesthesia or local anesthesia with intravenous sedation. We now routinely performing this procedure under local anesthesia only, as popularized by Lalonde and Wong [22]. We administer an injection of 20 mL 1 % lidocaine with 1:100,000 epinephrine buffered by 2 mL of 8.4 % sodium bicarbonate. By injecting 5 mL into the proximal, middle, and distal portions of the procedure site approximately 20–30 min prior to the procedure, full visualization of anatomic structures is possible while the patient remains comfortable. It also affords the convenience of allowing consumption of meals, which can be important for diabetics, and allows full cooperation in the operative suite. This technique should not be used in patients with an allergy to local anesthetics or patients with vascular pathology affecting the hand, fingers, or forearm. If anesthesia is requested by the patient or preferred by the surgeon, either sedation or general anesthesia may be used. For these cases, local anesthetic (typically a 1:1 mixture of 1 % lidocaine and 0.25 % bupivacaine without epinephrine) is injected after anesthesia but prior to incision, assuming no contraindications.

11.8.2 Positioning

The procedure is performed with the patient in the supine position with a hand table. A tourniquet is not typically applied with local anesthesia cases, but if no epinephrine is used, then a well-padded tourniquet is placed on the upper arm to aid in visualization during the procedure. The arm is abducted to 90° or to the patient's comfort, where it is sterilely prepped and draped. The following procedure is an adaptation of the procedure originally described by Chow [23], utilizing an extrabursal approach, to which he transitioned after its first description [20].

11.8.3 Landmarks

Figures 11.1 and 11.2 illustrate the preoperative marking of the incision sites.

11.8.4 Procedure

Figures 11.3, 11.4, 11.5, 11.6, 11.7, 11.8, 11.9, 11.10, 11.11, 11.12, 11.13, 11.14, 11.15, 11.16, 11.17, 11.18, 11.19, and 11.20 illustrate the rest of the procedure.

11.8.5 Postoperative Care

The patient is instructed to elevate the hand and to move the fingers into a fist 10 times every 2 h for the first 24 h, except while sleeping. The patient may remove the dressings on postoperative day 2 and shower normally, patting the hand dry, but the hand must not be soaked in standing water such as dishwater, a bathtub, or a swimming pool while the sutures are in place. Light activity is allowed when comfortable, but heavy activity should be avoided. The sutures are removed 7–10 days after surgery, when the incisions are healed. Activity is then progressed according to the tolerance of the patient.

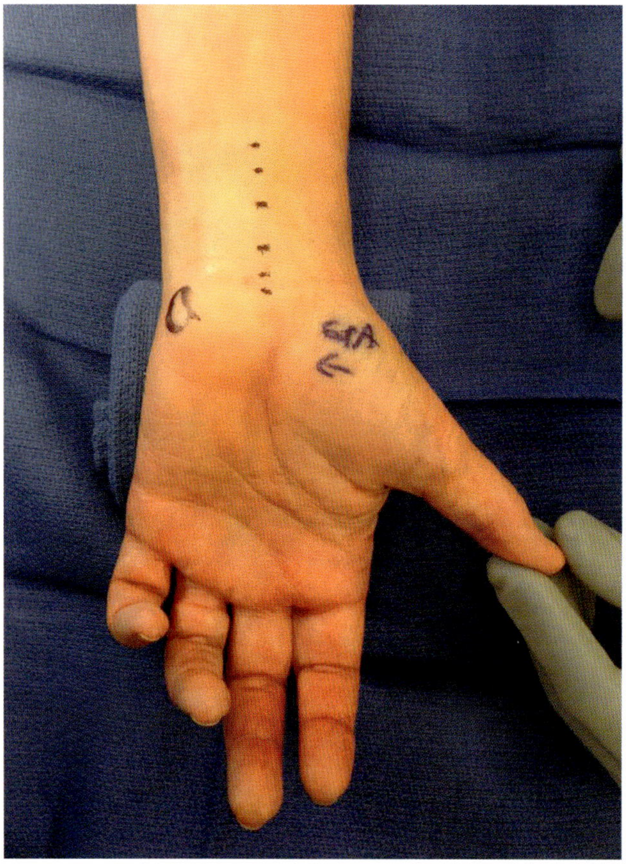

Fig. 11.1 We routinely mark the pisiform and draw the anticipated path of the median nerve (*dotted line*), which is directly beneath or slightly ulnar to the palmaris longus tendon (if present). The flexor carpi radialis should be easily palpable in most patients and serves as the radial extent of the median nerve's path, with the most ulnar aspect typically at the level of the flexor tendons

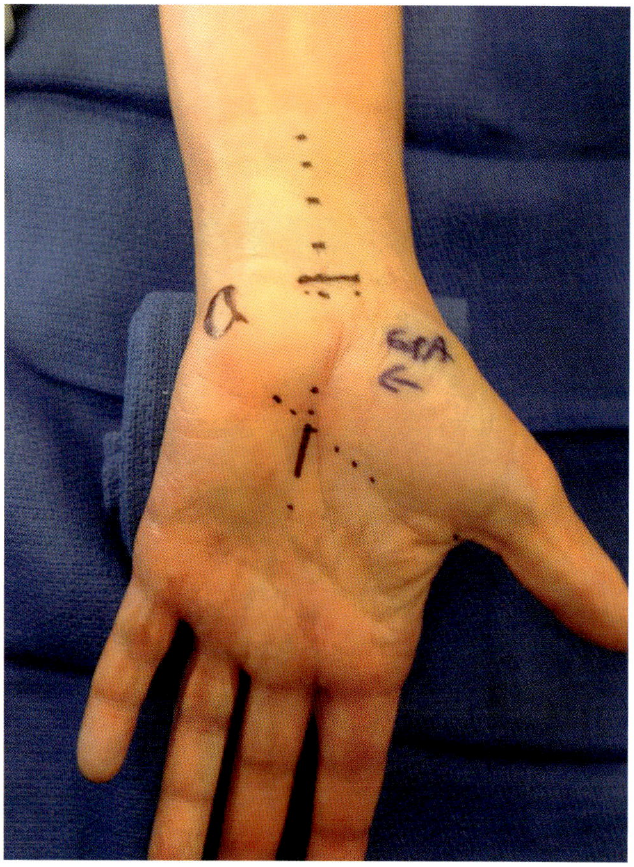

Fig. 11.2 Our proximal incision is centered to slightly radial over the median nerve. We choose to place it just proximal to the distal wrist flexion crease for patient comfort postoperatively. The distal, or palmar, incision is placed at the junction of a line connecting the fully radially abducted thumb and the hamate hook and a line drawn from the radial aspect of the ring finger

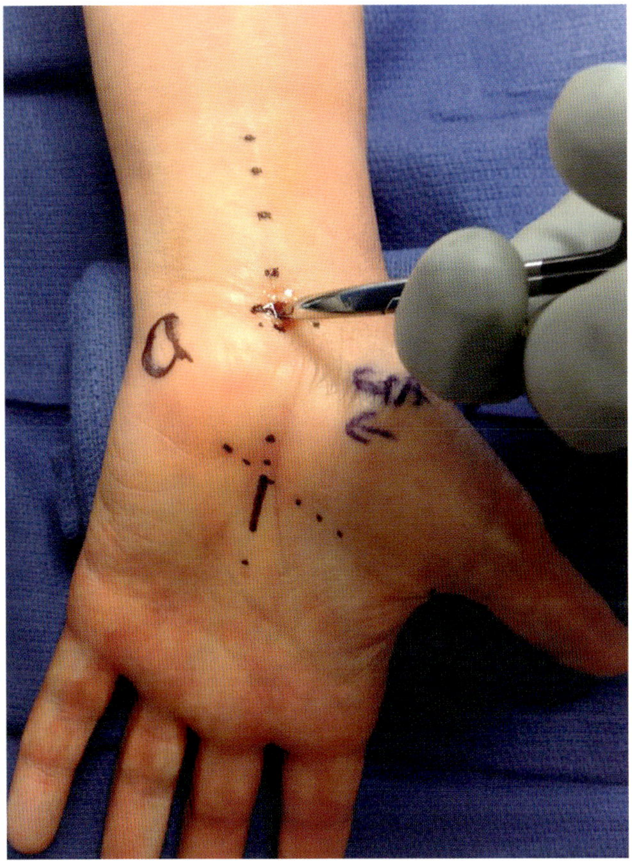

Fig. 11.3 Utilizing a #15 blade, the proximal skin is incised with dissection through the superficial tissue, in line with the median nerve, using a blunt tenotomy scissors to the antebrachial fascia

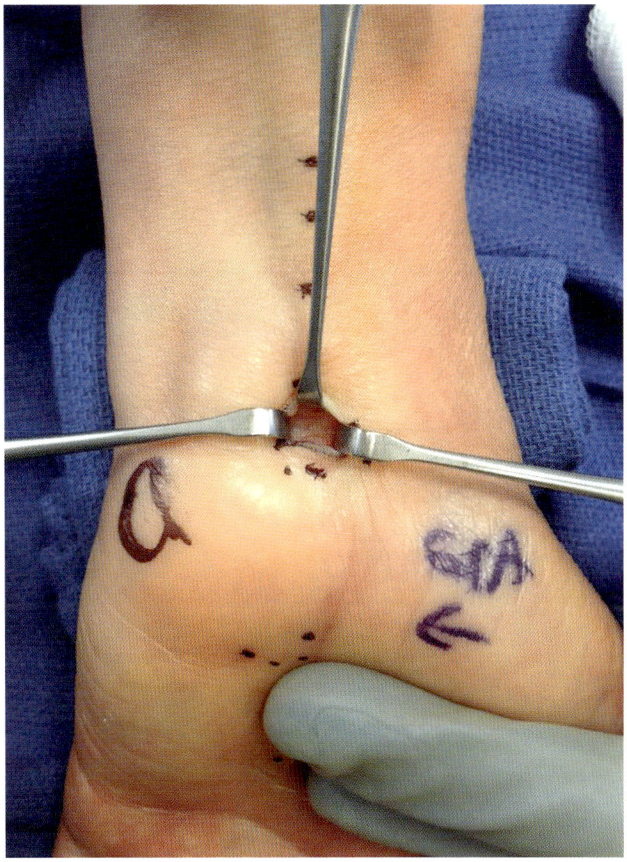

Fig. 11.4 Two medium smooth retractors aid the superficial retraction. The palmaris longus, if present, is retracted radially to protect the palmar cutaneous branch of the median nerve. A third retractor retracts the proximal skin to expose the antebrachial fascia for incision

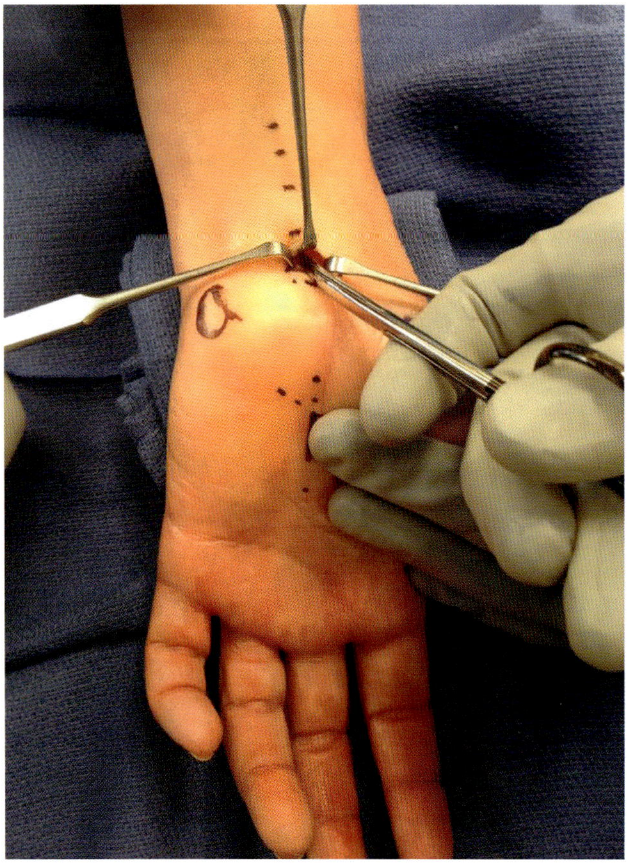

Fig. 11.5 A separate (deep) #15 blade is used to create an opening in the antebrachial fascia. The blunt tenotomy scissors are used to safely complete the proximal release of the antebrachial fascia. The scissors are directed proximally and slightly ulnarward, to protect the palmar cutaneous branch of the median nerve. The fascia is released for 2–3 cm

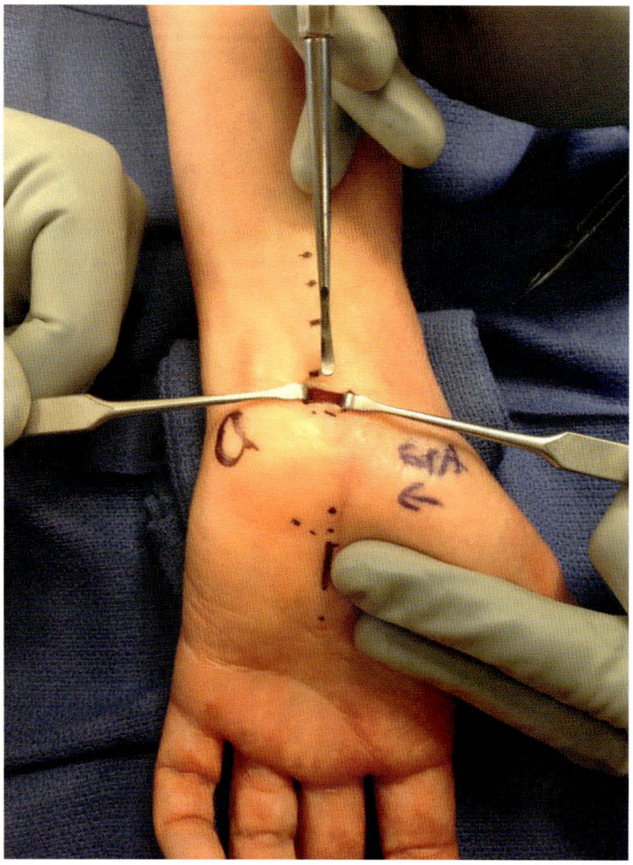

Fig. 11.6 A Chow elevator is inserted into the carpal tunnel at approximately a 45° angle through the proximal opening to create a path for the camera trocar. The elevator should be inserted carefully to avoid violation of the median nerve, which is easily visualized. The tip of the elevator is used to brush the undersurface of the transverse carpal ligament, creating a "washboard" sensation. Occasionally, in chronic cases of carpal tunnel syndrome, the transverse carpal ligament is adherent to the underlying contents, in which case the Chow elevator can be used to gently free the undersurface of the ligament

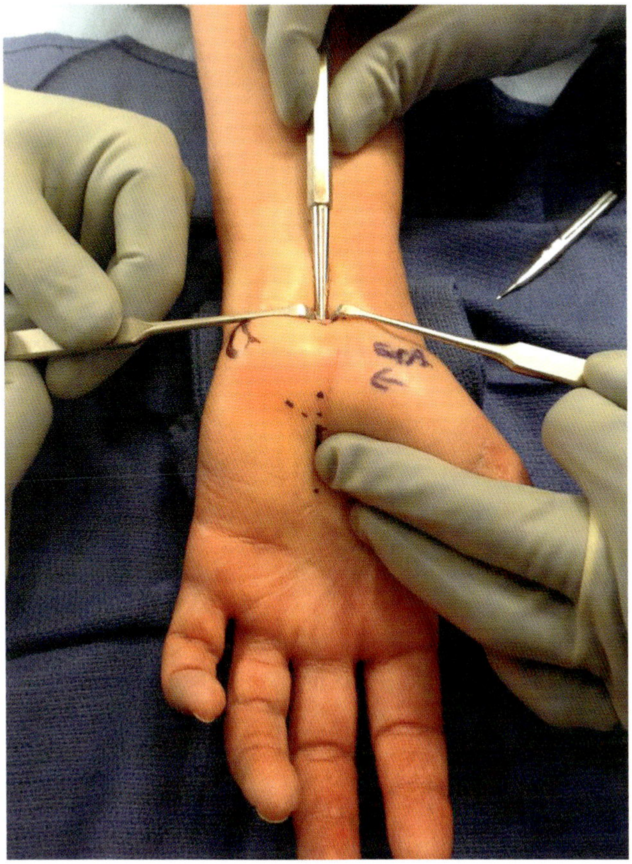

Fig. 11.7 Once the Chow elevator has traversed the extent of the ligament, the tip is palpable at the palmar incision. Palpation of the elevator tip distal to the previously marked incision should be carefully evaluated, as the superficial palmar arch will be in close proximity. Extending the wrist will displace the arch dorsally, protecting it from injury

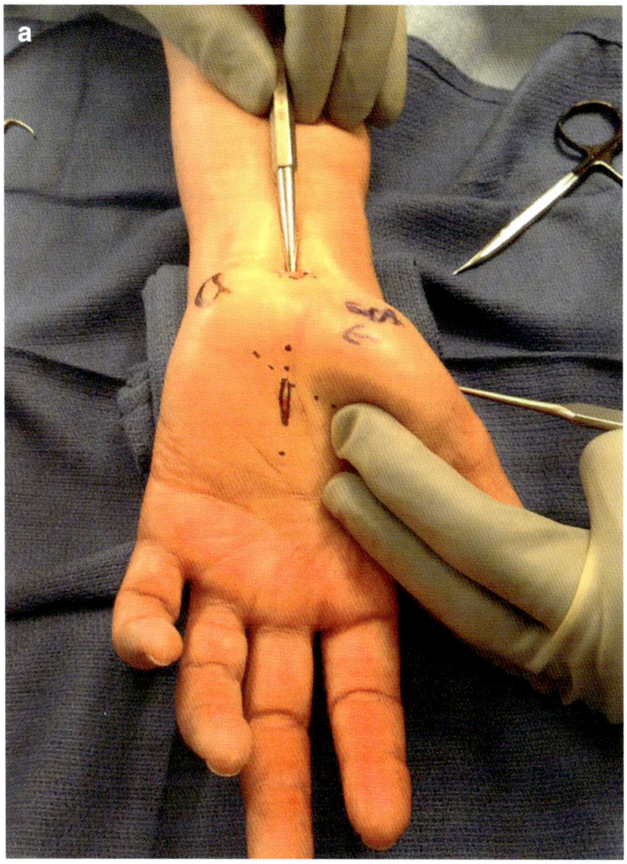

Fig. 11.8 (**a**–**c**) Distal incision is made with the "skin" #15 blade with dissection in line with palmar fascia, using the Stevens tenotomy scissors to create a path for the Chow elevator to be delivered through the distal surgical site. To decrease the chance of injury to the palmar arch, two medium smooth retractors aid in visualizing the tip of the Chow elevator as it is delivered distally

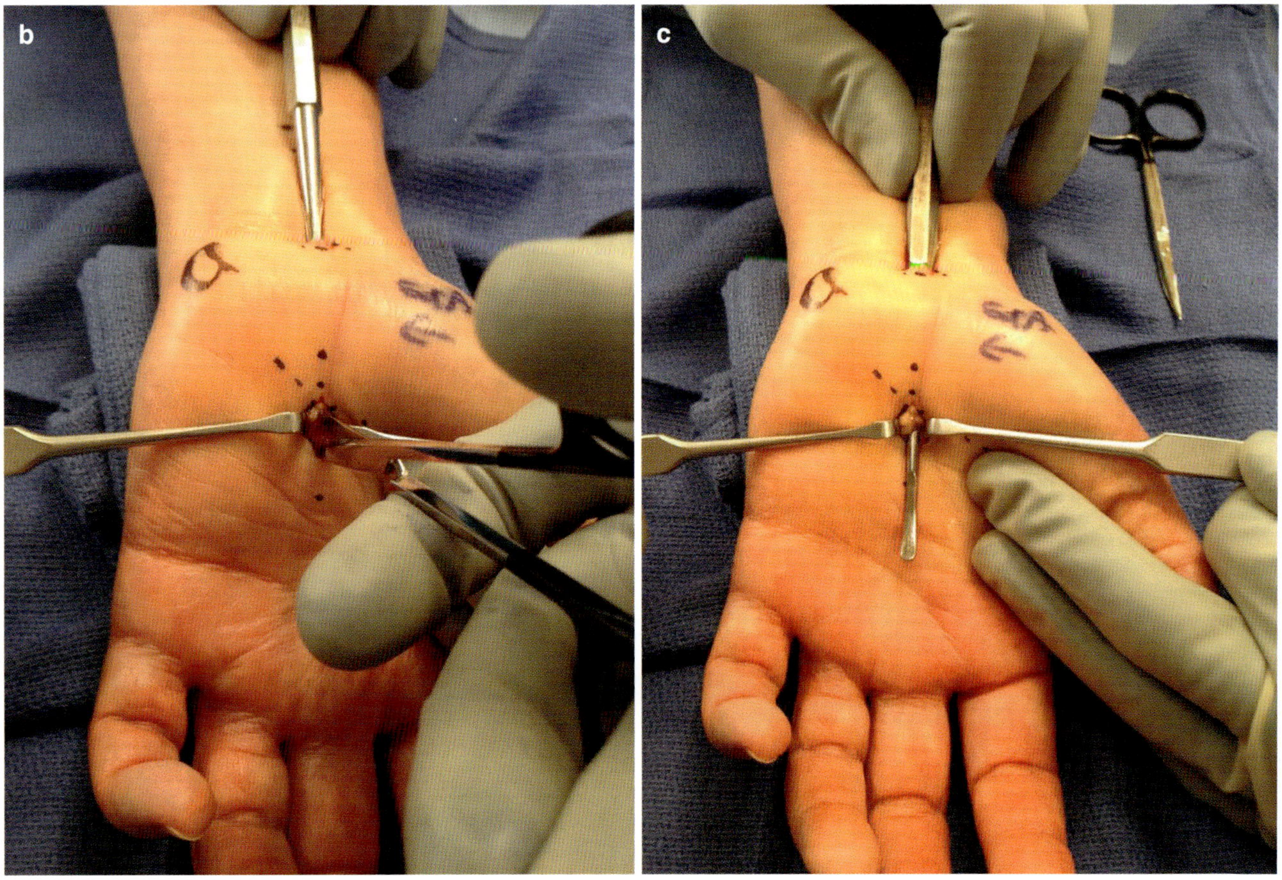

Fig. 11.8 (continued)

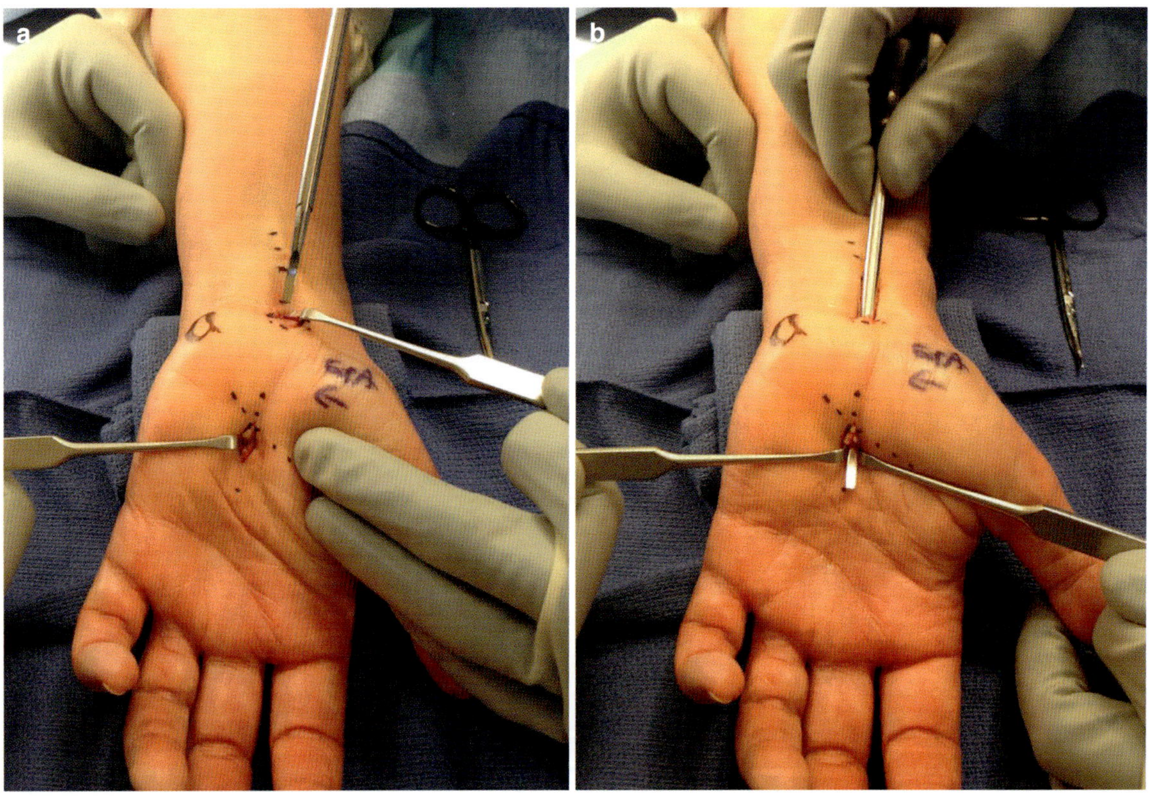

Fig. 11.9 (**a**, **b**) Leaving one medium smooth retractor in the distal site and moving one to the proximal site, the slotted camera trocar with obturator is inserted beneath the transverse carpal ligament, using the obturator tip to "scrub" the undersurface of the ligament as previously done with the Chow elevator. As the obturator tip approaches the palmar incision, both medium smooth retractors protect the palmar arch by aiding its delivery

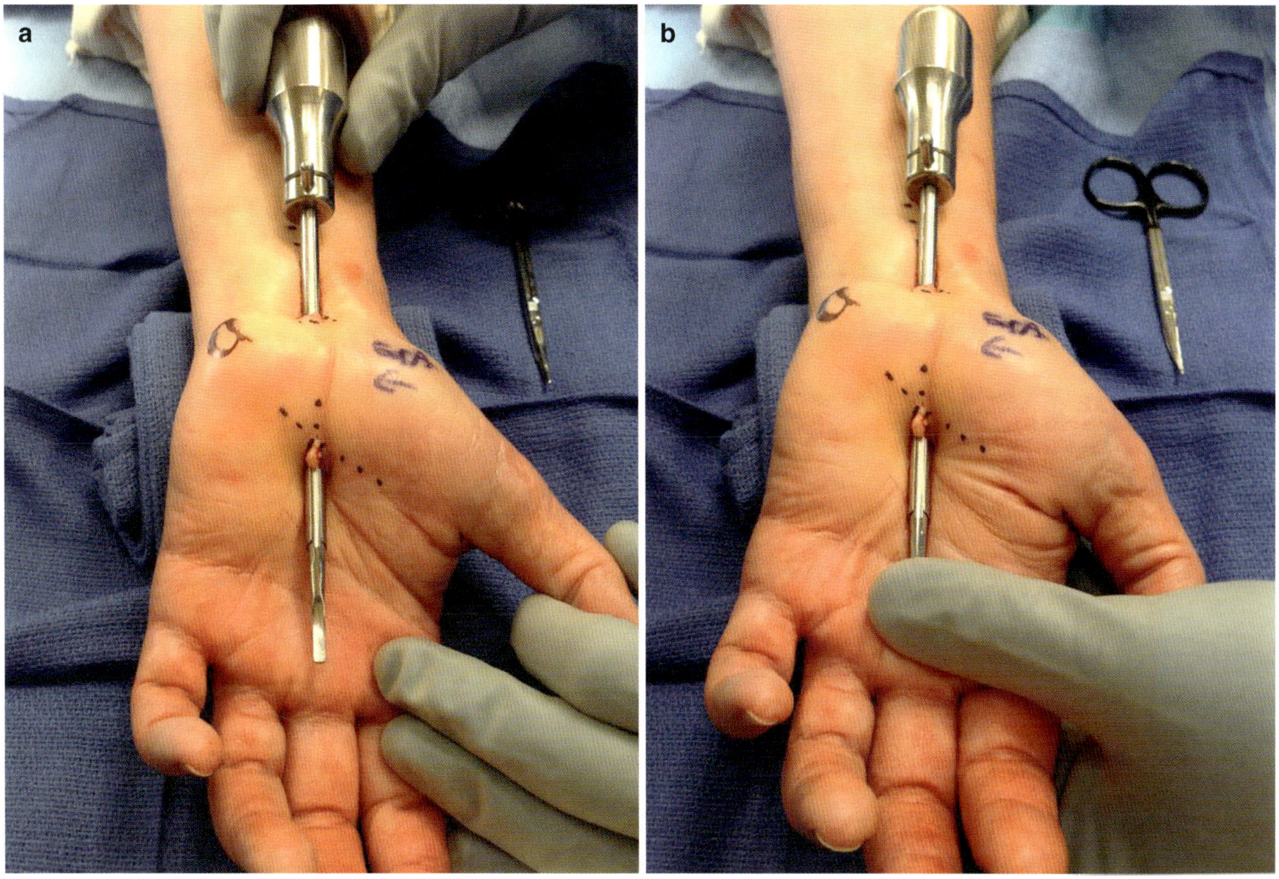

Fig. 11.10 Once the trocar has been delivered through the palmar incision (**a**), a thumb should be placed in the curved end of the obturator (**b**) to control the rotation of the trocar while the hand is positioned on the endoscopic platform

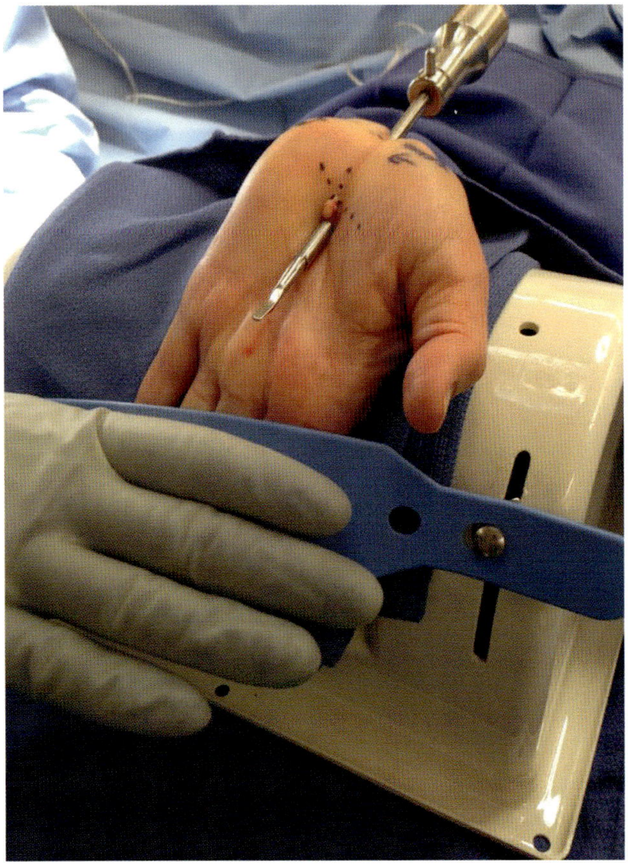

Fig. 11.11 The extremity is placed on the endoscopic platform with the elbow flexed to approximately 45° and the wrist extended to 70° (or the patient's comfort level). A strap is placed over the fingers to allow instrument insertion through each end of the trocar

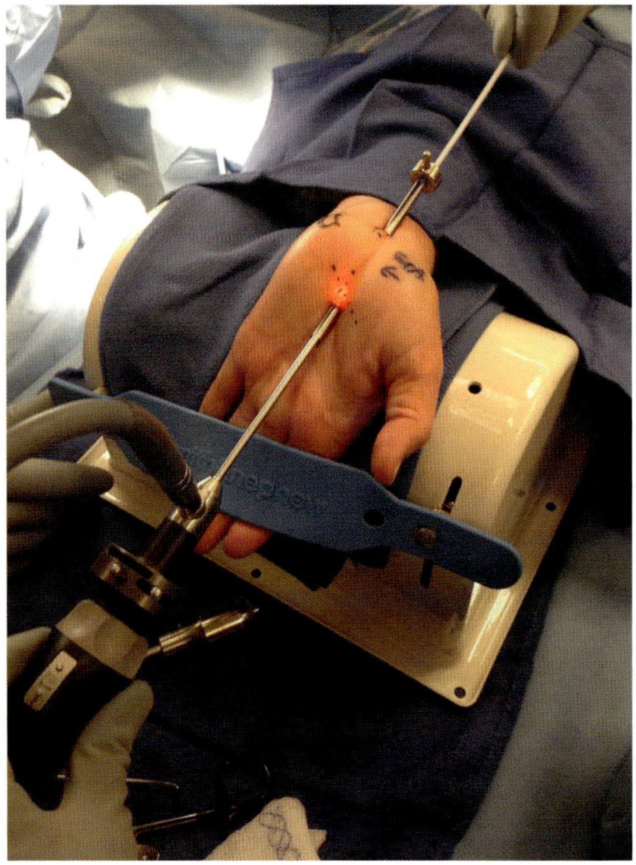

Fig. 11.12 A 30° endoscope is inserted through the distal end of the trocar and a sterile Q-tip is rotated through the proximal end to clear any adipose tissue or debris from the undersurface of the ligament and the trocar opening, for excellent visualization. As the Q-tip is inserted, it should be rotated radially to avoid pulling any stray epineurium from the recurrent branch of the median nerve into the trocar opening

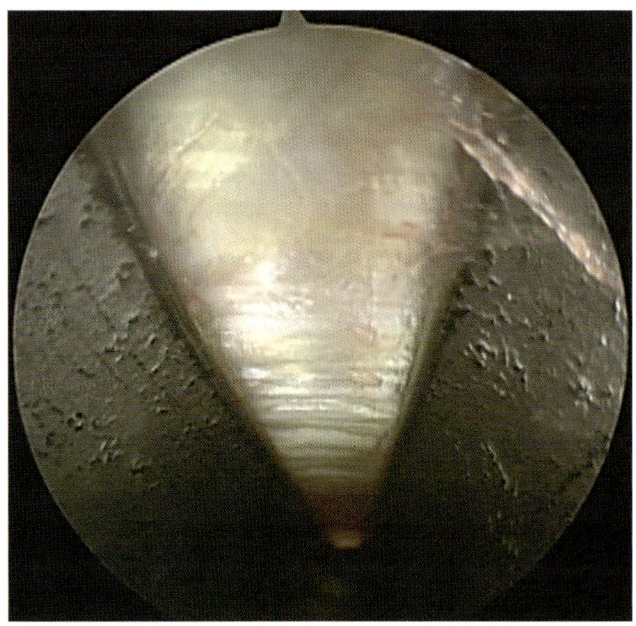

Fig. 11.13 Endoscopic view after the Q-tip has been passed, showing excellent visualization of the undersurface of the transverse carpal ligament. If there is any question of aberrant structures, the endoscopic technique should be converted to an open procedure, as the recurrent branch of the median nerve piercing the transverse ligament has been reported [24]

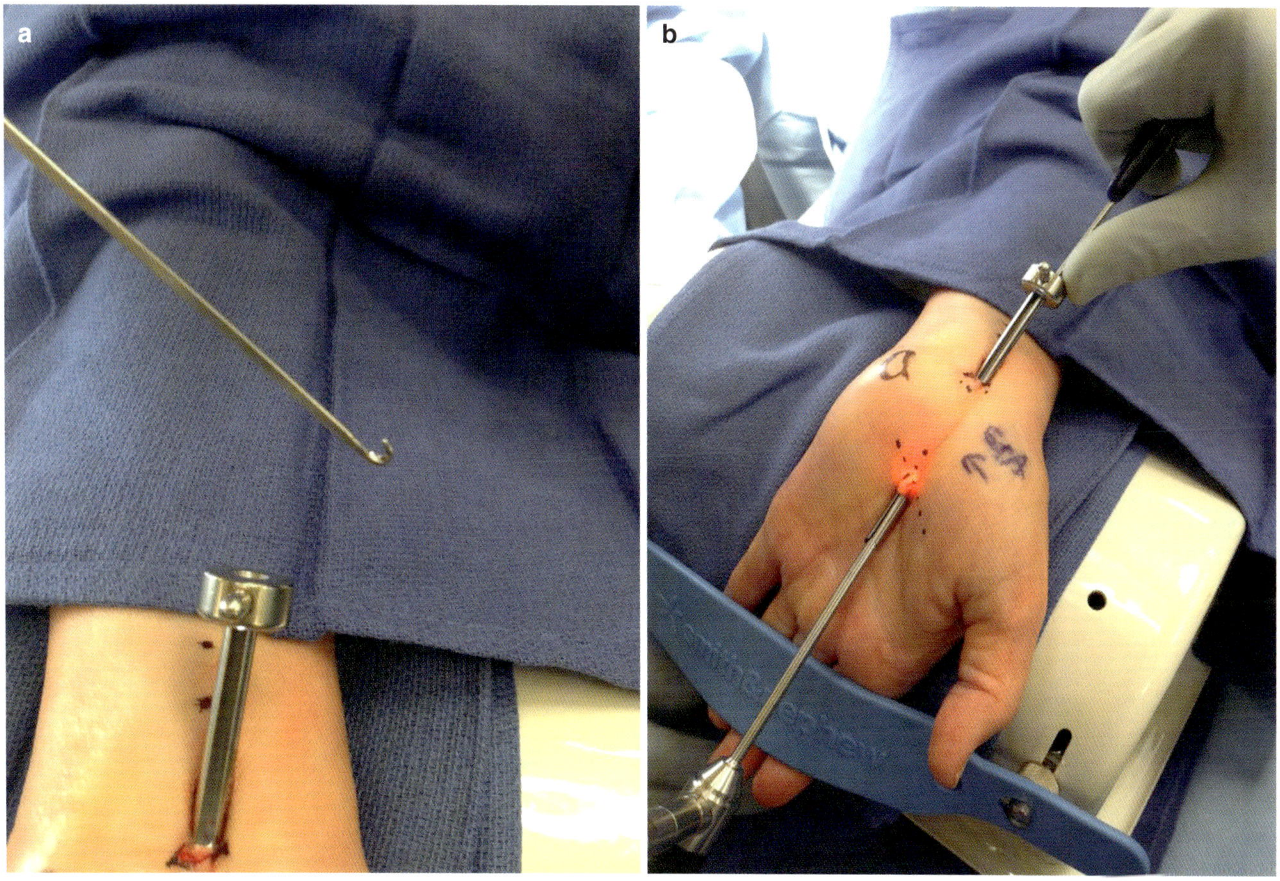

Fig. 11.14 (**a**, **b**) A reverse cutting endoscopic knife is then inserted under direct visualization with the endoscope, to divide the ligament from distal to proximal. We choose to use a knife with a smooth hook to engage the distal extent of the ligament, but other options are available. To further protect the median nerve, the surgeon's hand should be pulled radially in order to move the knife blade ulnarly, and the knife should be ulnarly rotated so that the division within the trocar occurs on the ulnar border of the slit. If any resistance is encountered, the knife can be removed to ensure that the recurrent branch of the median nerve is not endangered

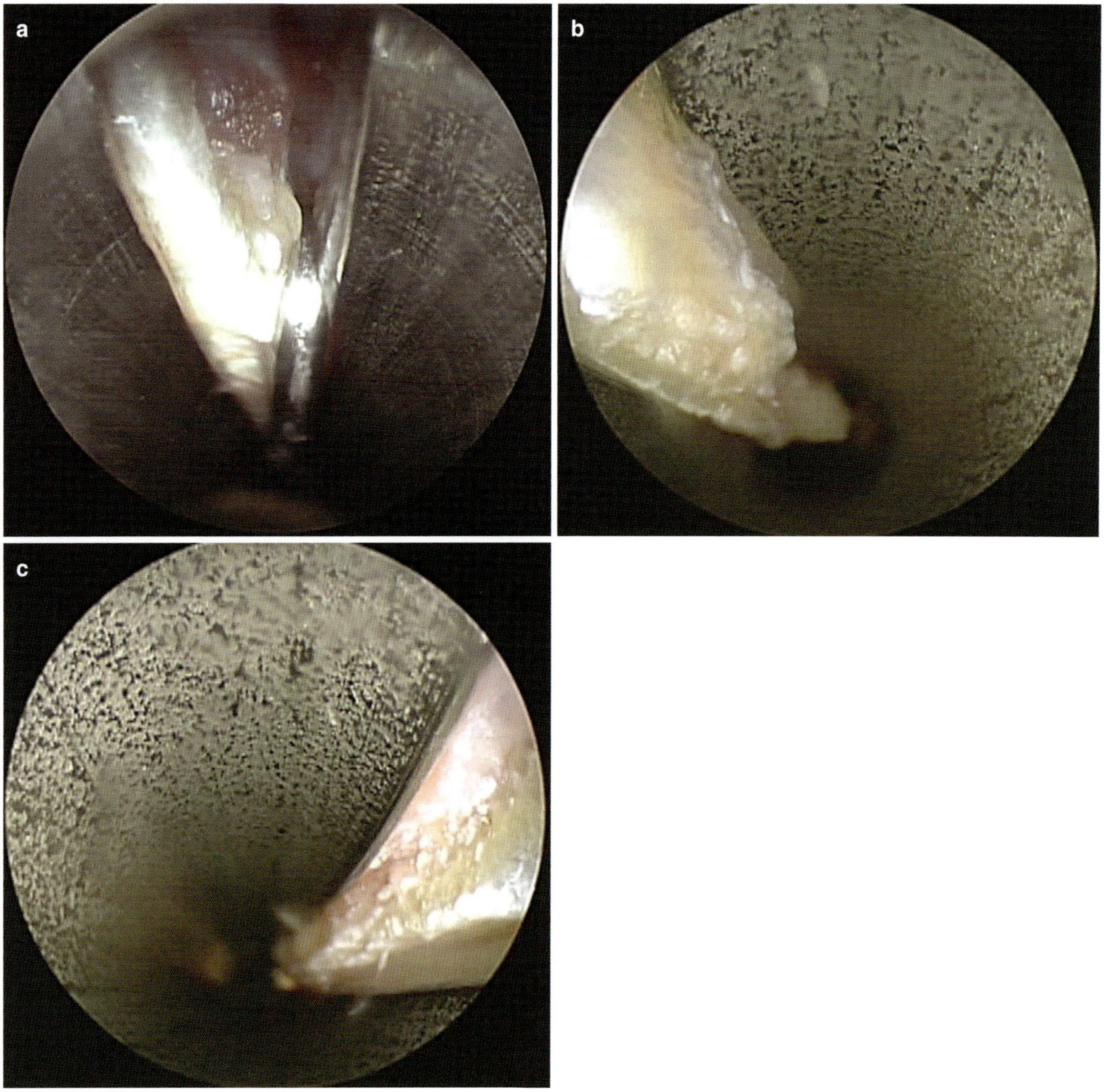

Fig. 11.15 The ligament is divided smoothly, staying on the ulnar side of the slotted trocar (**a**). After division, the trocar can be slightly rotated radially and ulnarly (**b**, **c**) to identify the sectioned edges of the ligament

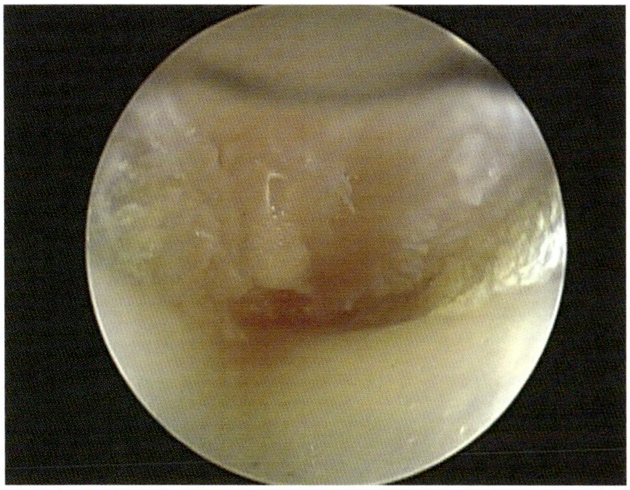

Fig. 11.16 After successful division of the ligament, the slotted trocar is removed, leaving the endoscope in place. This figure demonstrates the view without the trocar; the transected edges of the ligament can be seen. The median nerve is seen as the structure at the bottom of the endoscopic view

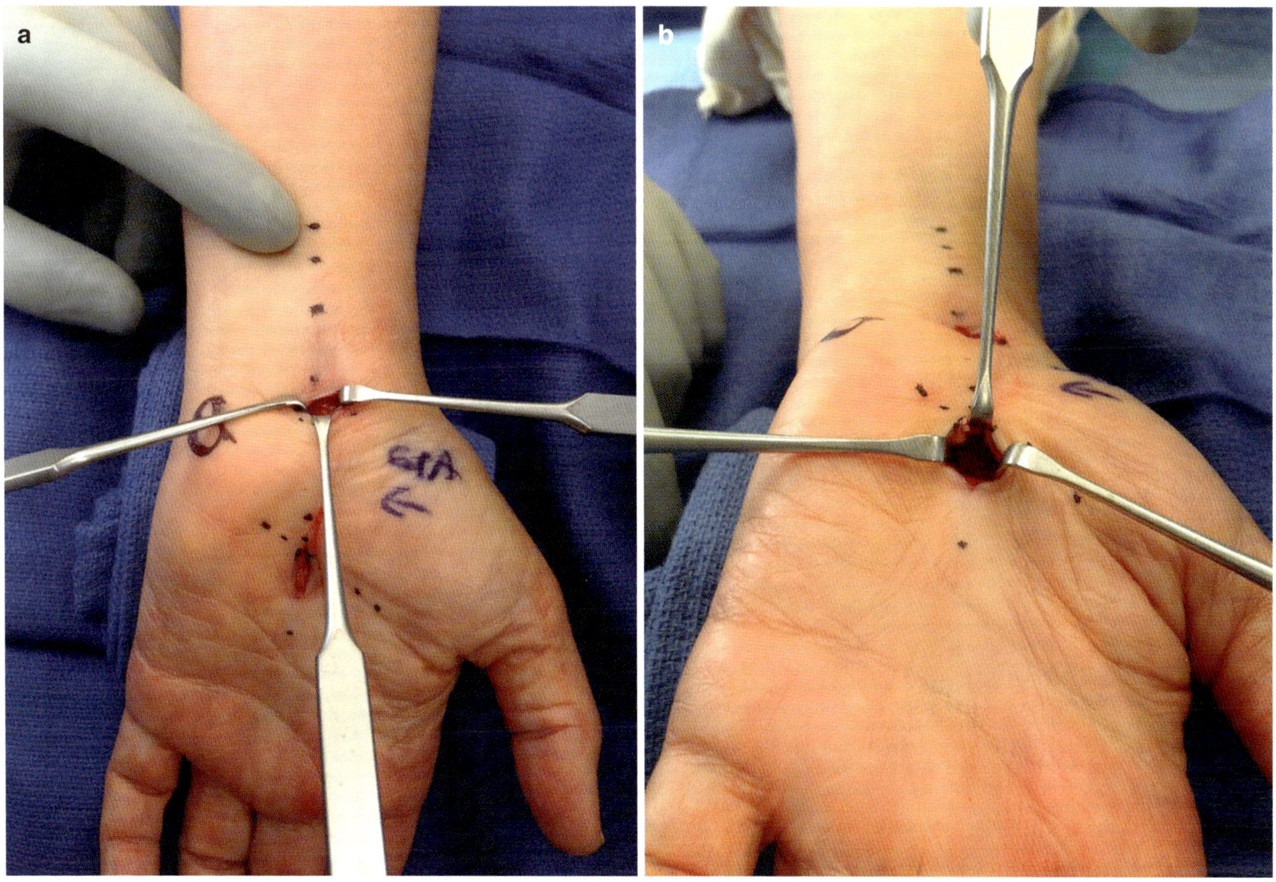

Fig. 11.17 After removal of the endoscope and trocar, the proximal (**a**) and distal (**b**) sites are inspected for successful division of the ligament

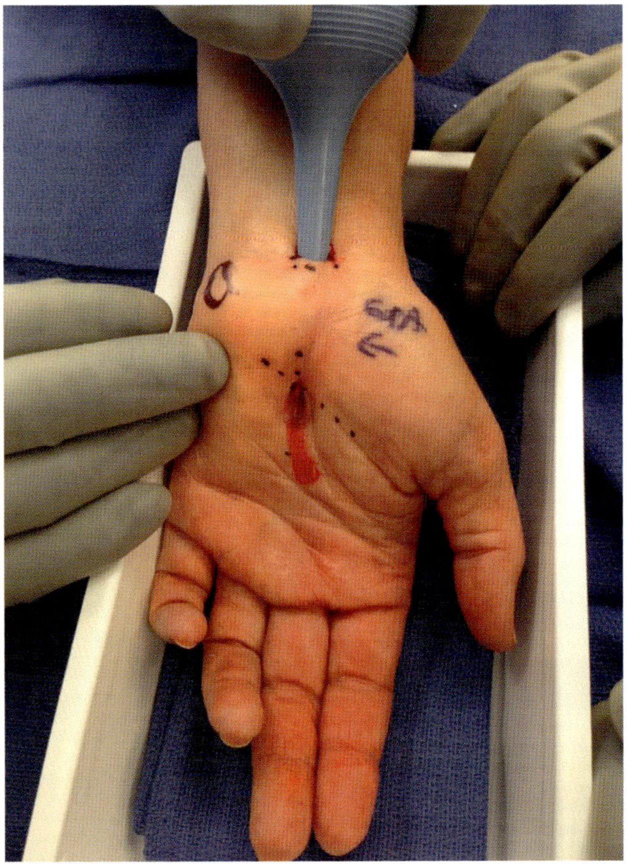

Fig. 11.18 The surgical site is copiously irrigated with a bulb syringe delivering warm normal saline from proximal to distal. Care is taken not to release the bulb within the wound, protecting the median nerve

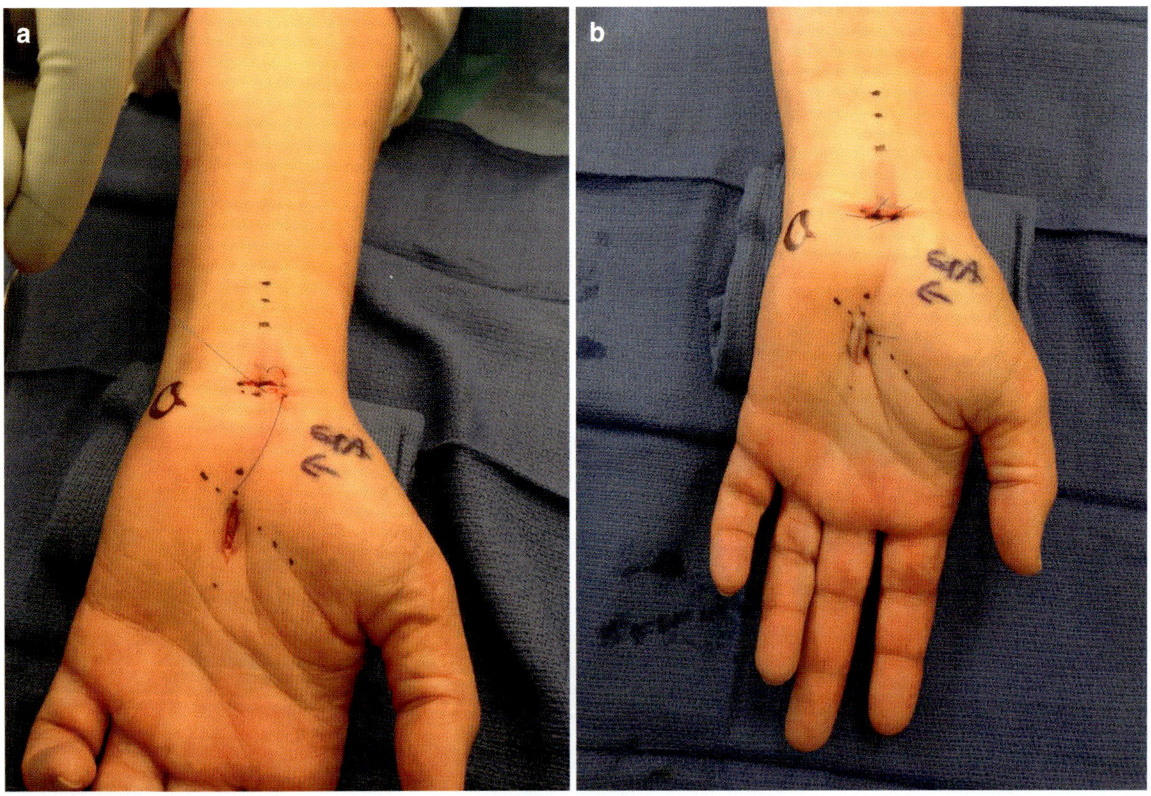

Fig. 11.19 (**a**, **b**) The surgical wounds are closed with a nonabsorbable suture, such as 4-0 Prolene™, in a horizontal mattress fashion

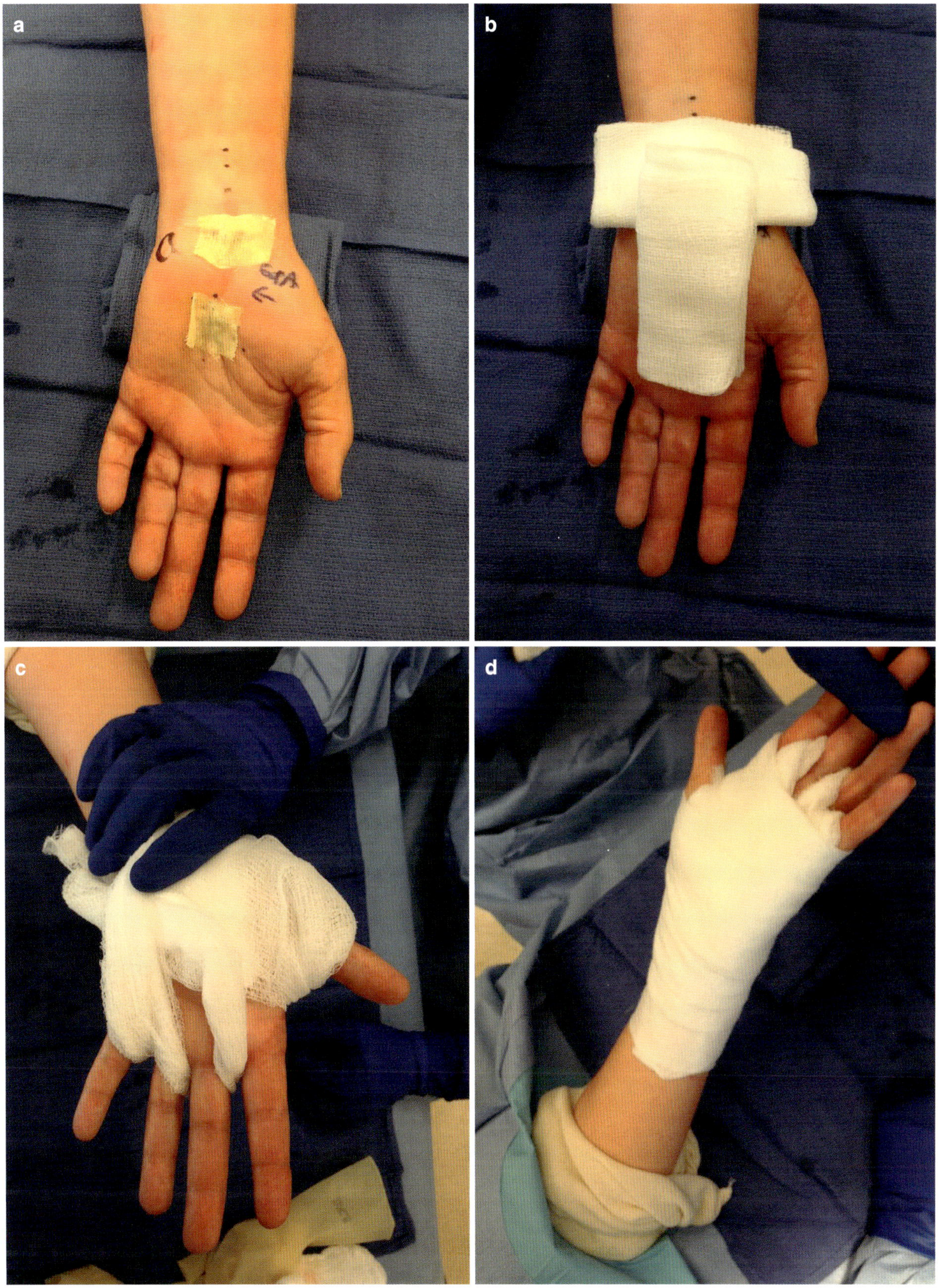

Fig. 11.20 (**a–e**) A sterile, soft dressing is applied, consisting of nonadherent gauze, 4×4 gauze over the wound and between adjacent digits, cotton or gauze sterile under wrap, and a compressive overwrap

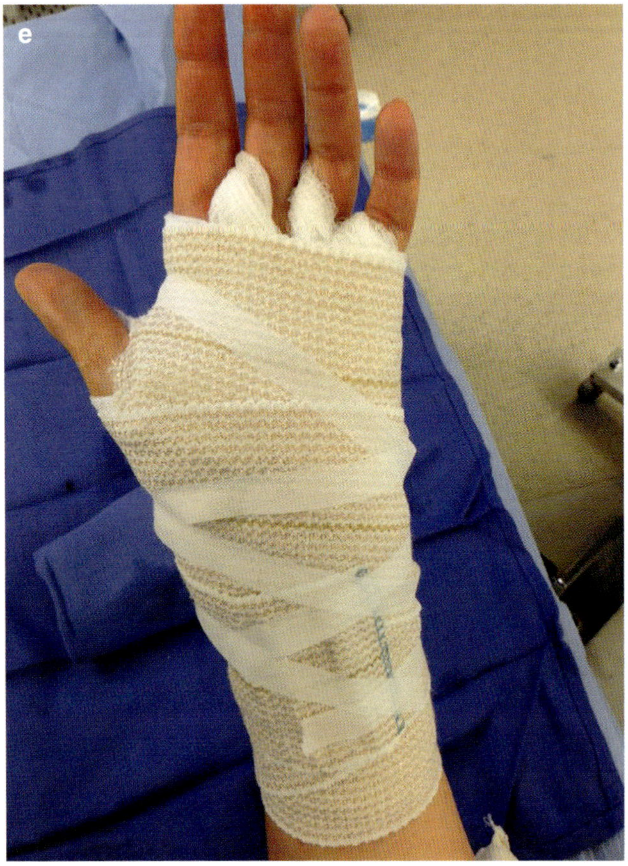

Fig. 11.20 (continued)

References

1. Paget J. Lectures on surgical pathology. Philadelphia: Lindsay & Babiston; 1990. p. 1842–54.
2. Palmer DH, Paulson JC, Lane-Larsen CL, Peulen VK, Olson JD. Endoscopic carpal tunnel release: a comparison of two techniques with open release. Arthroscopy. 1993;9:498–508.
3. Mosier BA, Hughes TB. Recurrent carpal tunnel syndrome. Hand Clin. 2013;29:427–34.
4. Hansen TB, Majeed HG. Endoscopic carpal tunnel release. Hand Clin. 2014;30:47–53.
5. Ibrahim I, Khan WS, Goddard N, Smitham P. Carpal tunnel syndrome: a review of the recent literature. Open Orthop J. 2012;6: 69–76.
6. Chow JCY. Endoscopic release of the carpal ligament for carpal tunnel syndrome: 22-month clinical result. Arthroscopy. 1990;6: 288–96.
7. Dorwart BB. Carpal tunnel syndrome: a review. Semin Arthritis Rheum. 1984;14:134–40.
8. Nathan PA, Keniston RC. Carpal tunnel syndrome and its relation to general physical condition. Hand Clin. 1993;9:253.
9. Chen CH, Wu T, Sun JS, Lin WH, Chen CY. Unusual causes of carpal tunnel syndrome: space occupying lesions. J Hand Surg Eur Vol. 2012;37:14–9.
10. Kulman KA. Sensitivity and specificity of carpal tunnel syndrome sign. Am J Phys Med Rehabil. 1997;76:451–7.
11. Naranjo A, Ojeda S, Mendoza D, Francisco F, Quevedo JC, Erausquin C. What is the diagnostic value of ultrasonography compared to physical evaluation in patients with idiopathic carpal tunnel syndrome? Clin Exp Rheumatol. 2007;25:853–9.
12. Amirfeyz R, Gozzard C, Leslie IJ. Hand evaluation test for assessment of carpal tunnel syndrome. J Hand Surg Br. 2005;30:361–4.
13. Gellman H, Chandler DR, Petrasek J, Sie I, Adkins R, Waters RC. Carpal tunnel syndrome in paraplegic patients. J Bone Joint Surg Am. 1988;70:517–9.
14. Durkan JA. A new diagnostic test for carpal tunnel syndrome. J Bone Joint Surg Am. 1991;73:535–8.
15. Durkan JA. The carpal-compression test. An instrumented device for diagnosing carpal tunnel syndrome. Orthop Rev. 1994;23: 522–5.
16. Knibb W. Health economics in surgery. Surgery. 2009;27:389–93.
17. Nathan PA, Keniston RC, Meadows KD. Predictive value of nerve conduction measurements at the carpal tunnel. Muscle Nerve. 1993;16:1377–82.
18. Witt JC, Hentz JG, Stevens JC. Carpal tunnel syndrome with normal nerve conduction studies. Muscle Nerve. 2004;29:515–22.
19. Green DP. Diagnostic and therapeutic value of carpal tunnel injection. J Hand Surg Am. 1984;9:850–4.
20. Chow JCY. The Chow technique of endoscopic release of the carpal ligament for carpal tunnel syndrome: four years of clinical results. Arthroscopy. 1993;9:301–14.
21. Botte MJ. Controversies in carpal tunnel syndrome. Instr Course Lect. 2008;57:199–212.
22. Lalonde DH, Wong A. Dosage of local anesthesia in wide awake hand surgery. J Hand Surg Am. 2012;38:2025–8.
23. Chow JCY. Endoscopic carpal tunnel release: two portal technique. Hand Clin. 1994;10:637–44.
24. Wolf AW, Packard S, Chow JCY. Transligamentous motor branch of the median nerve discovered during endoscopically assisted carpal tunnel release. Arthroscopy. 1993;9:222–3.

12 Endoscopic Flap Design and Harvesting

Yoko Katsuragi-Tomioka and Masahiro Nakagawa

The use of endoscopes has achieved general acceptance in most areas of surgery. Plastic surgery was not one of the earliest specialties to incorporate endoscopic surgical techniques, but because of its overriding demand for smaller incisions, its use has become popular in recent decades. After Teimourian and Kroll [1] reported the use of a subcutaneous endoscope in suction lipectomy in 1984, indications in plastic surgery increased rapidly, especially in the 1990s.

The first indication for the use of an endoscope in plastic surgery was for the release of the carpal ligament [2], for forehead or brow lifts [3, 4], for breast surgery [5, 6], and for abdominoplasties [7, 8]. Surgical endoscopy expanded rapidly, and various flaps began to be harvested with endoscopic assistance. Harvesting of the omentum [9, 10], the jejunal free flap [11, 12], the latissimus dorsi [13–16], the rectus abdominis [17, 18], and the gracilis [19–21] were all reported in the mid-1990s. Indications are still expanding, such as in cranioplasties [22] and maxillofacial traumas [23–25].

Because intramuscular dissection is necessary to harvest perforator flaps, accomplishing the whole procedure under endoscopy is not easy, but the findings obtained by an endoscopic approach surely help the surgeon to make intraoperative decisions. These techniques enable minimum sacrifice of the donor site, precise design, less stress on the surgeon, and an educational opportunity for the assistants and audience.

It is well known that the perforator of the anterolateral thigh (ALT) flap is often located at the midpoint of the anterior superior iliac spine and the lateral margin of the patella [26], but of course this location varies. When harvesting a large flap, this uncertainty is not a problem, as the perforator will be included anyway, but when it comes to harvesting a small flap, there is a risk that the initial design will not include the perforator (Fig. 12.1).

The classic approach was to confirm the design after making a long incision and locating the perforator, or to harvest a large flap and trim it afterwards. By providing added information about the exact location of the perforator, endoscopes make it possible to avoid extra skin incision or extra tissue harvesting (Fig. 12.2).

Y. Katsuragi-Tomioka, MD (✉) • M. Nakagawa, MD, PhD
Division of Plastic and Reconstructive Surgery,
Shizuoka Cancer Center Hospital,
Shimonagakubo 1007, Naga-izumi, Shizuoka 411-8777, Japan
e-mail: yoko-prs@umin.ac.jp; m.nakagawa@scchr.jp

E. Raposio (ed.), *Atlas of Endoscopic Plastic Surgery*, DOI 10.1007/978-3-319-19461-5_12

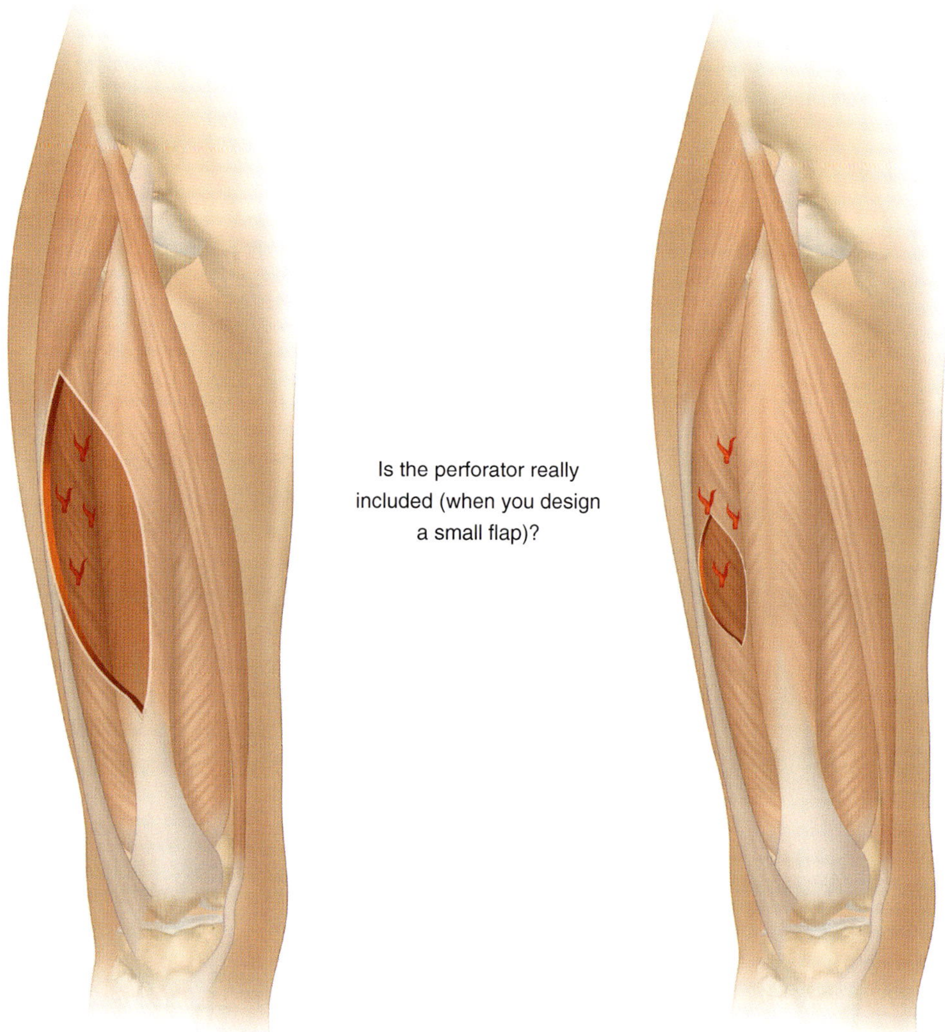

Fig. 12.1 Large flaps would include the perforators anyway. On the other hand, it is difficult to design small flaps

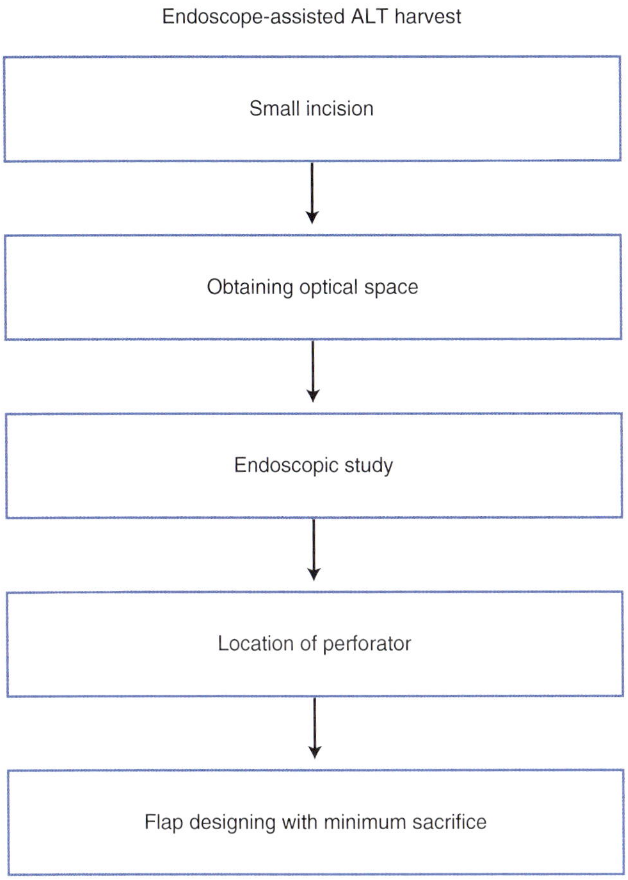

Fig. 12.2 Steps of harvesting anterolateral thigh (ALT) flaps using an endoscope. By obtaining information about the exact location of the perforator, the endoscope makes it possible to avoid extra skin incision or extra tissue harvesting

12.1 Training

Handling of endoscopes requires some training, for which we recommend using suitable animal models. Perforator flaps of pigs are a preferable animal model, considering their size and the structure of the subcutaneous tissue. For the example shown in Fig. 12.3, a female Yorkshire pig weighing 35 kg was used at our Animal Laboratory in compliance with the *Guide for the Care and Use of Laboratory Animals for Institutions of the Governing Agency* published by the Japanese Ministry of Health, Labor and Welfare. A 2-cm skin incision is first made in the thigh of the pig, and the cavity for the endoscopic camera is made using manual retractors.

Then a standard 10-mm, 0°-angle endoscopic camera is put into the subcutaneous layer (Fig. 12.4).

Standard surgical endoscopic instruments such as scissors, dissectors, and monopole coagulators are used to dissect the subcutaneous layer and to cut the tissue surrounding the perforator (Fig. 12.5).

The subcutaneous tissue is loose, so dissectors are applied first to make this layer honeycomb-like (Fig. 12.6); then scissors are used to cut the remaining fibrous tissue (Fig. 12.7).

Tissues including vessels are coagulated by monopole diathermy. An aspirator at the incision helps to clear the misty view. Though the skin incision is short, the surgeon and the assistants can see everything more closely and much more clearly because the lens of the camera has a wide angle and high magnification, so it is not difficult to find the perforator in the subcutaneous tissue. After detecting the perforator and marking its location, the flap is designed and the skin incision is performed to harvest the flap (Figs. 12.8, 12.9, and 12.10).

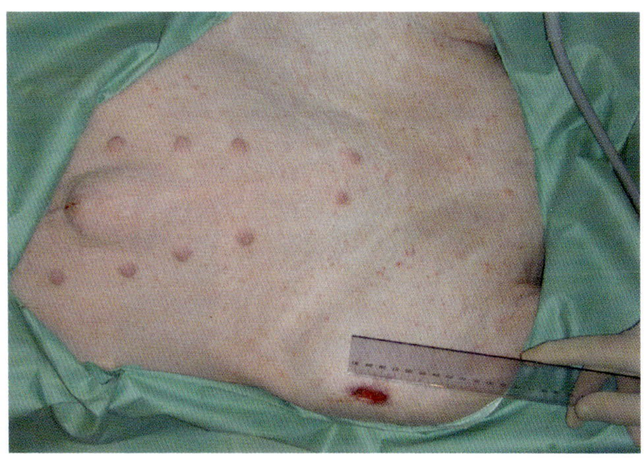

Fig. 12.3 An incision (2 cm in length) made in the thigh of a pig for endoscopic training

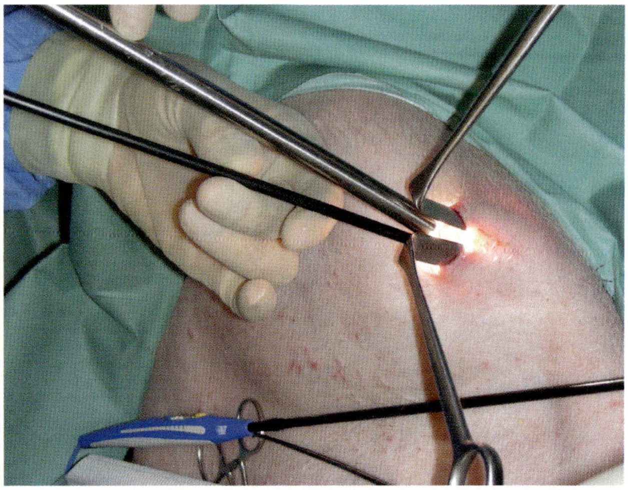

Fig. 12.4 Two retractors are inserted to obtain optic space. A standard 10-mm, 0°-angle endoscopic camera is put into the subcutaneous layer

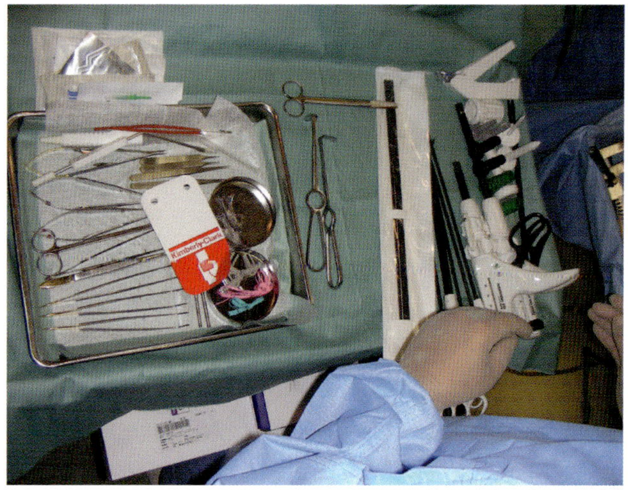

Fig. 12.5 Standard surgical endoscopic instruments, including scissors, dissectors, and monopole coagulators

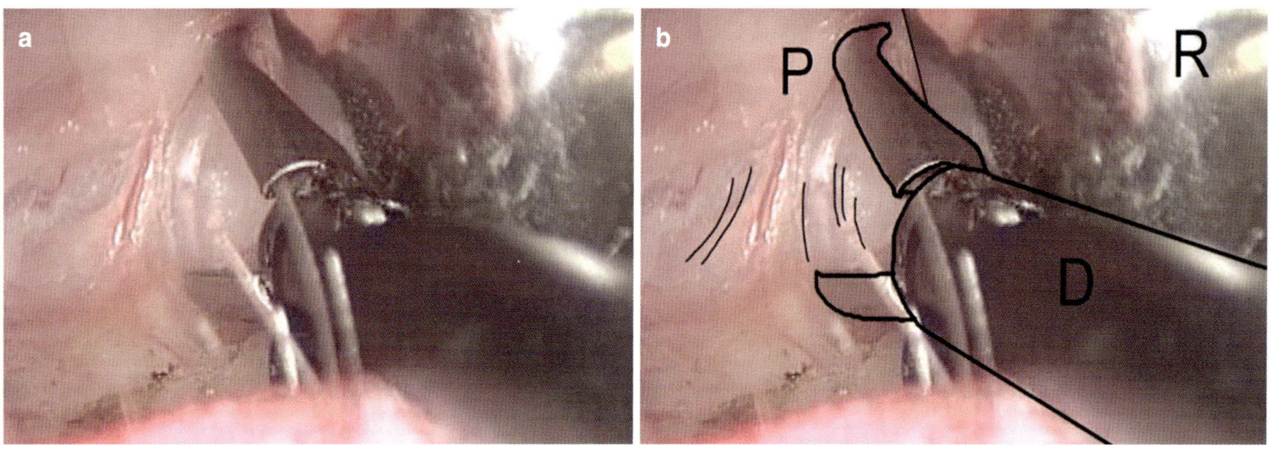

Fig. 12.6 (**a**, **b**) The loose subcutaneous tissue is first dissected to become honeycomb-like. *D* dissector, *R* retractor, *P* perforator

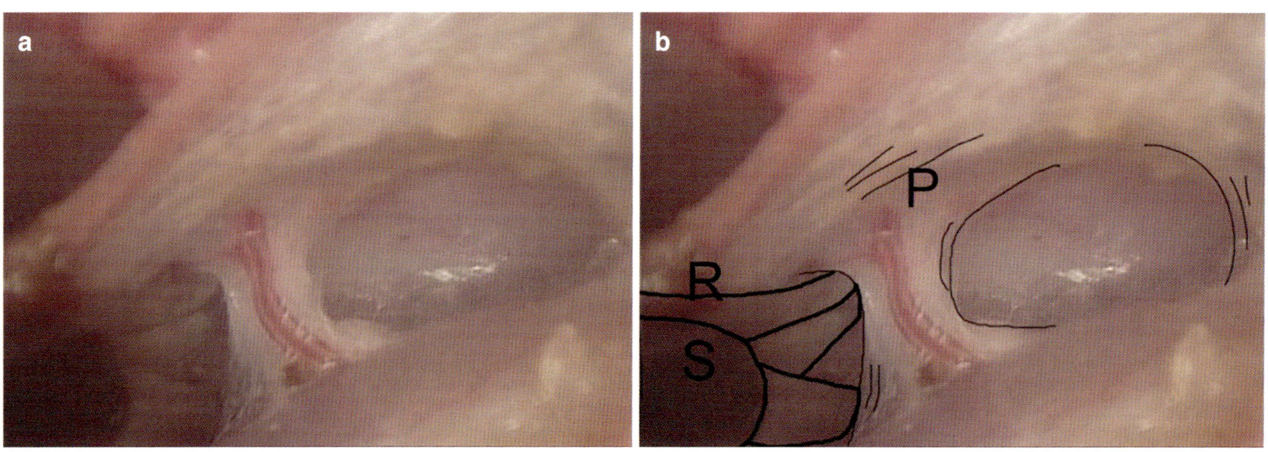

Fig. 12.7 (**a**, **b**) Scissors cutting the remaining fibrous tissue. *P* perforator, *R* retractor, *S* scissors

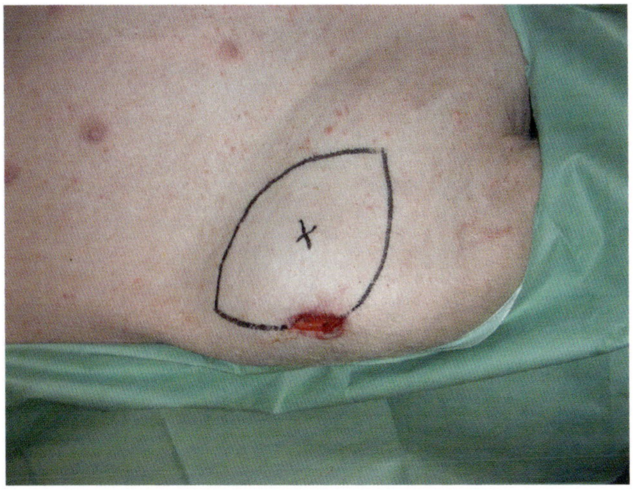

Fig. 12.8 After the location of the perforator has been confirmed, the flap is designed

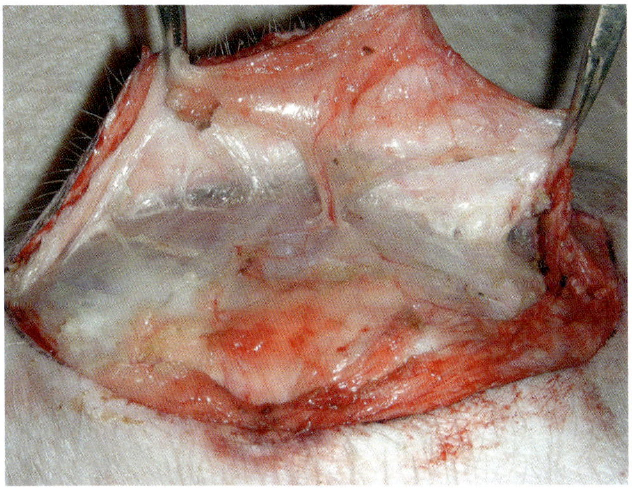

Fig. 12.9 Endoscopic dissection can isolate the perforator

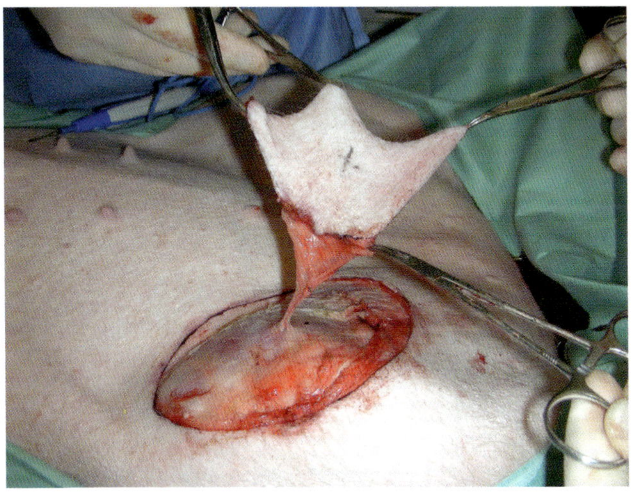

Fig. 12.10 The perforator flap is harvested

12.2 Surgical Technique

After a brief survey of the perforators with a hand-held Doppler, a 2-cm skin incision is made at the anterior aspect of the thigh (Fig. 12.11).

This incision can be made either medial or lateral to the line through the anterior superior iliac spine and the lateral margin of the patella, but the lateral approach does not require the procedure to cross the septum to find the musculocutaneous perforators arising from the vastus lateralis (Fig. 12.12).

Subcutaneous tissue is dissected with two retractors to the femoral fascia. An incision is made through the fascia, and the edges of the fascia are clamped by a Kocher or mosquito clamp (Fig. 12.13).

After dissection of the subfascial layer under direct vision, one retractor is inserted to pull up the fascia and one to push down the rectus femoralis or the lateral vastus muscle to obtain an optical cavity (Fig. 12.14).

A 3-mm, 0°-angle endoscopic camera (Fig. 12.15) is inserted into this working space, and microdissecting forceps are placed to perform subfascial dissection.

The procedure is performed under endoscopy, which enables the surgeons to find even the smallest perforators with large magnification. The video monitor also allows the assistants to have the same view as the surgeons (Fig. 12.16).

Though the subfascial tissue is loose, the first view would look like Fig. 12.17.

As was done in the training procedure, microdissecting forceps are applied to detach the loose areolar tissue (Fig. 12.18).

Normal scissors are then applied to isolate the perforator (Fig. 12.19).

The high magnification of the endoscope provides a fine view of even the smallest perforators (Fig. 12.20).

Once the perforators are detected, their location is marked using the transillumination from the light source (Fig. 12.21).

Flap design is then confirmed, and the flap is harvested with the usual technique.

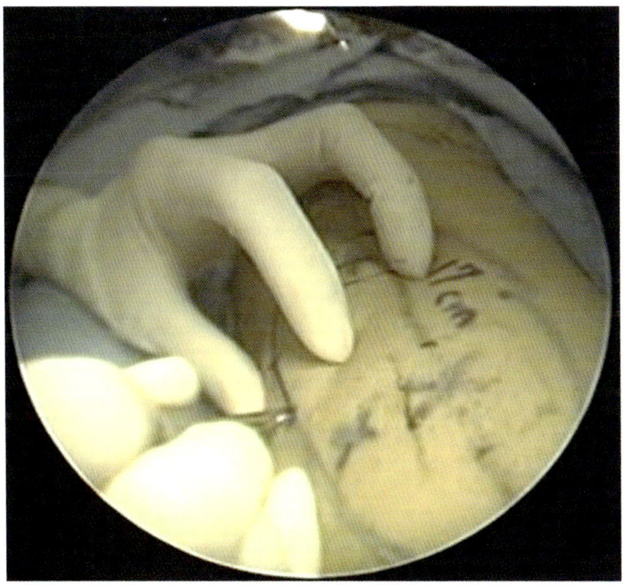

Fig. 12.11 Skin incision to the lateral aspect of the thigh

Fig. 12.12 Schema of endoscopic harvesting of an ALT flap

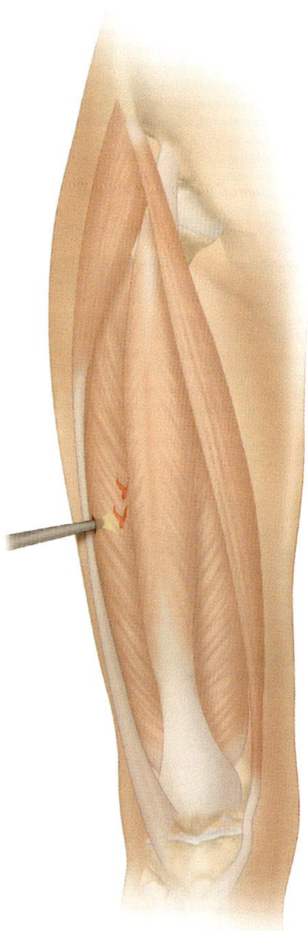

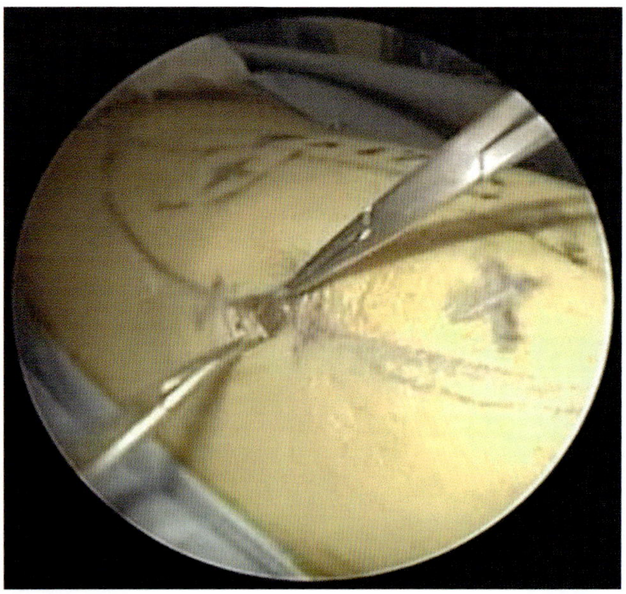

Fig. 12.13 After dissection of the subcutaneous tissue with two retractors, the femoral fascia is incised and the edge is clamped by Kocher or mosquito clamps

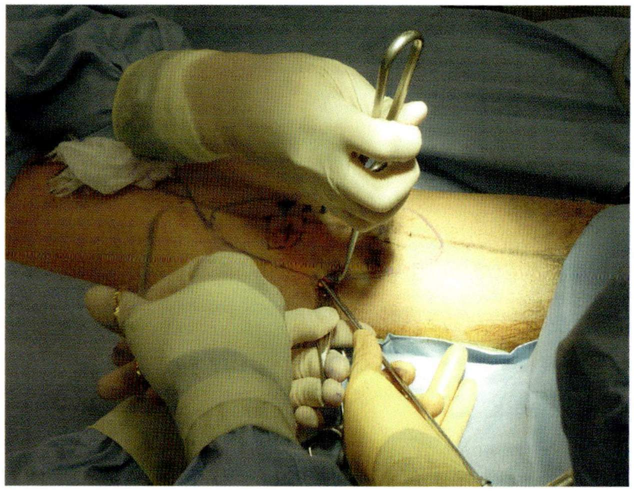

Fig. 12.14 One retractor is inserted to pull up the fascia to obtain an optical cavity

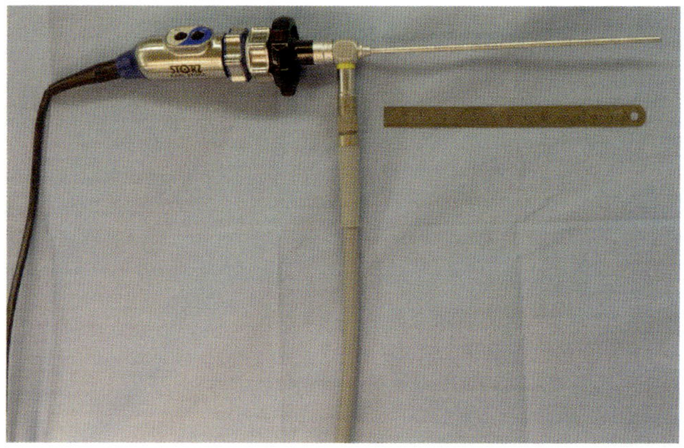

Fig. 12.15 A 3-mm, 0°-angle endoscopic camera

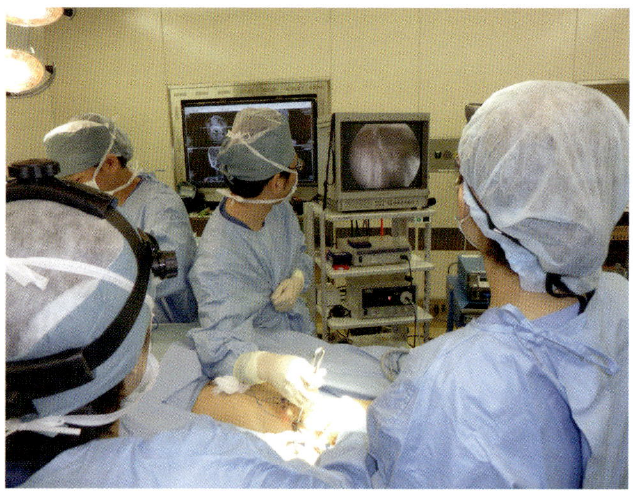

Fig. 12.16 The video provides both the surgeon and the assistants with a wide-angle, high-magnification view

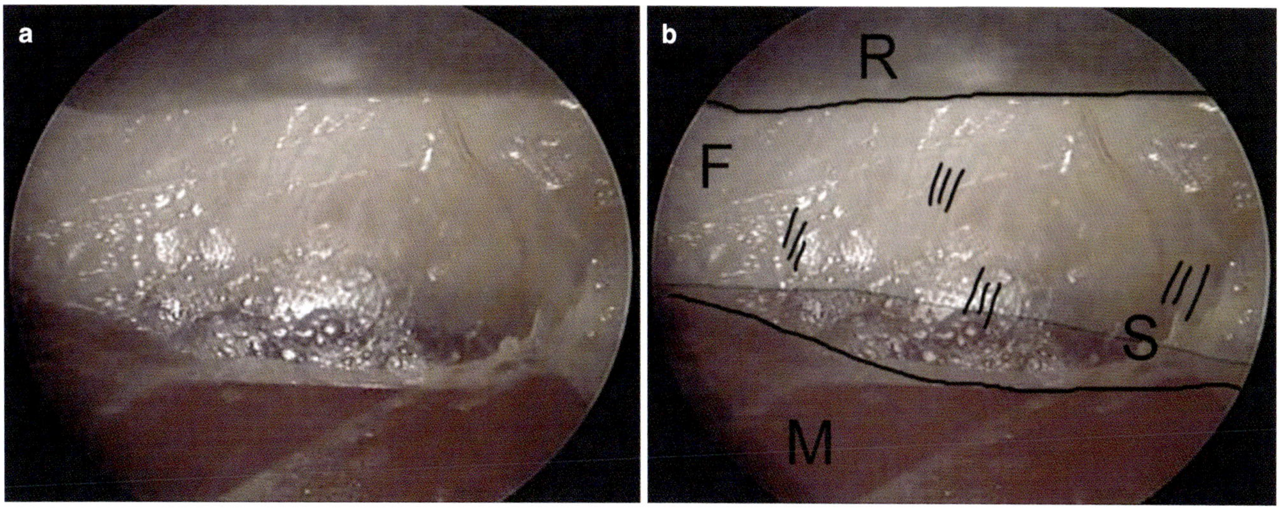

Fig. 12.17 (**a**, **b**) The view from the camera in the subfascial layer above the vastus lateralis. *F* fascia, *M* vastus lateralis muscle, *R* retractor, *S* loose areolar tissue of the subfascial layer

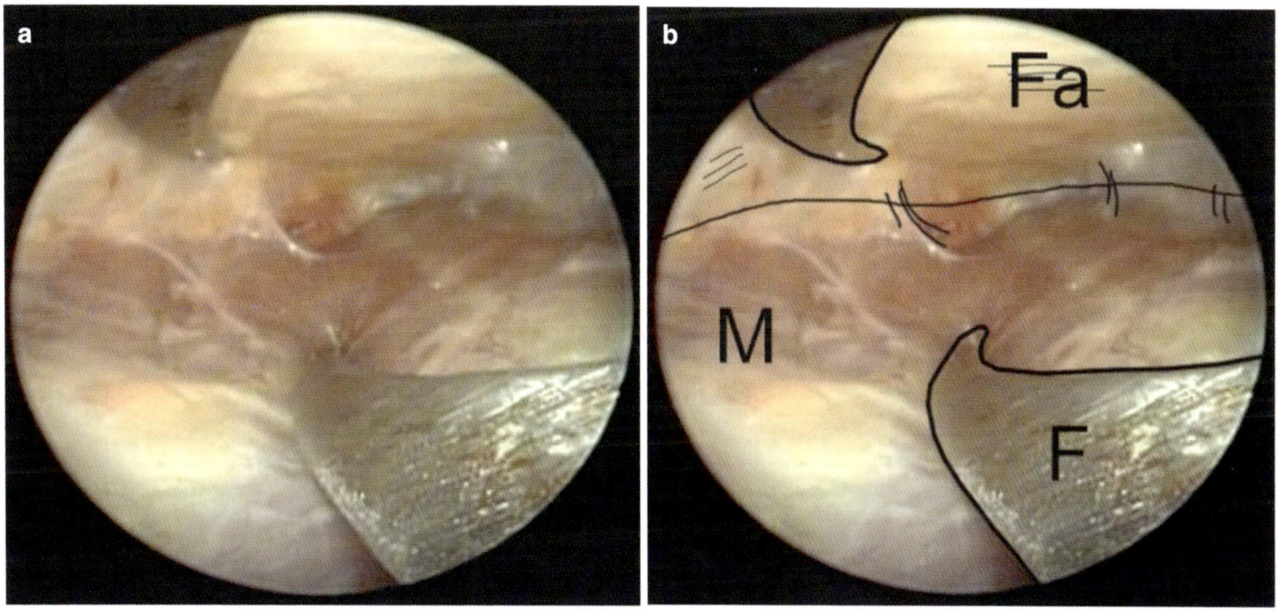

Fig. 12.18 (**a**, **b**) Microdissecting forceps are used to detach the loose areolar tissue. *F* forceps, *Fa* fascia, *M* vastus lateralis muscle

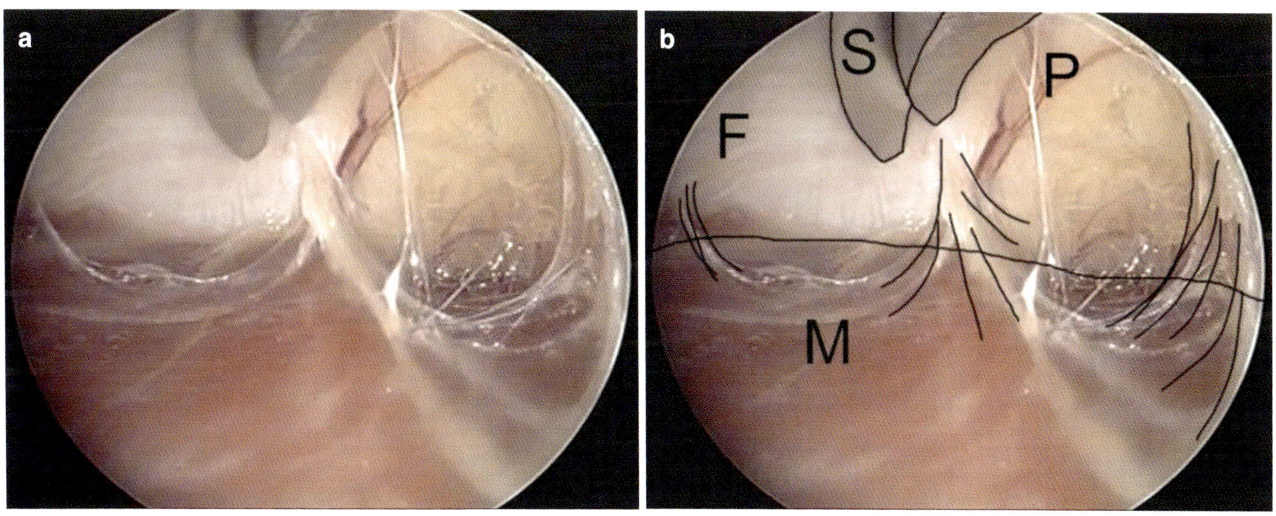

Fig. 12.19 (**a**, **b**) Normal scissors are then used to isolate the perforator. *F* fascia, *M* vastus lateralis muscle, *P* perforator, *S* scissors

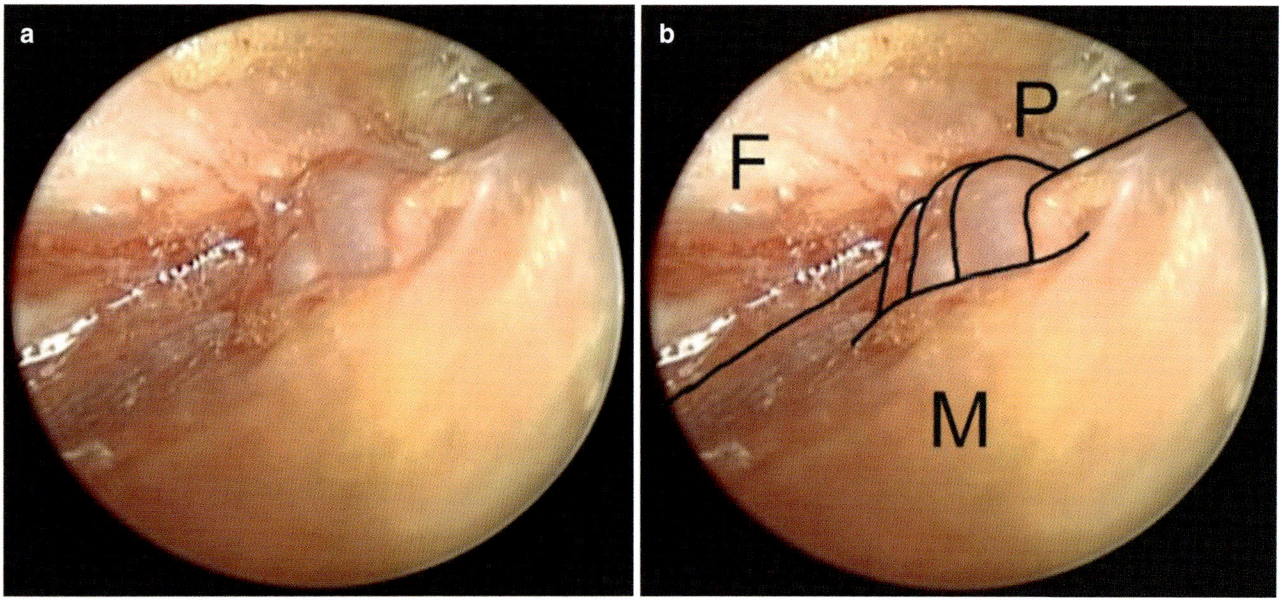

Fig. 12.20 (**a**, **b**) The isolated perforator arising from the muscle. On video, even the smallest perforators with their pulsation can be seen under the high-magnification view. *F* fascia, *M* vastus lateralis muscle, *P* perforator

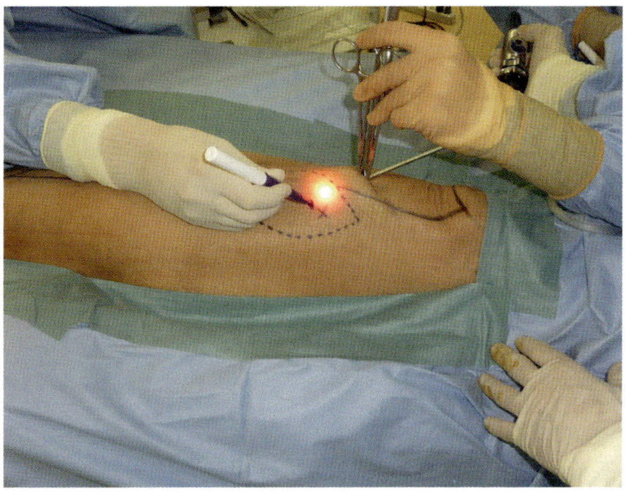

Fig. 12.21 The location of the perforator is marked by transillumination from the light source, and then the flap is designed [27]

12.3 Results

Endoscopy is useful to ensure the location of the perforator, leading to precise flap design. The flap can be harvested without any extra skin incision or extra tissue harvesting. Endoscopic findings minimize donor morbidity because there is no need to make the flap larger than the defect in order to "be sure" that the perforator is included (Fig. 12.22).

Endoscopy is especially useful when small flaps are needed or when the exact location of the perforator is important. The technique is also useful for deep inferior epigastric artery perforator flaps, and has the potential to be furthered applied to other perforator flaps.

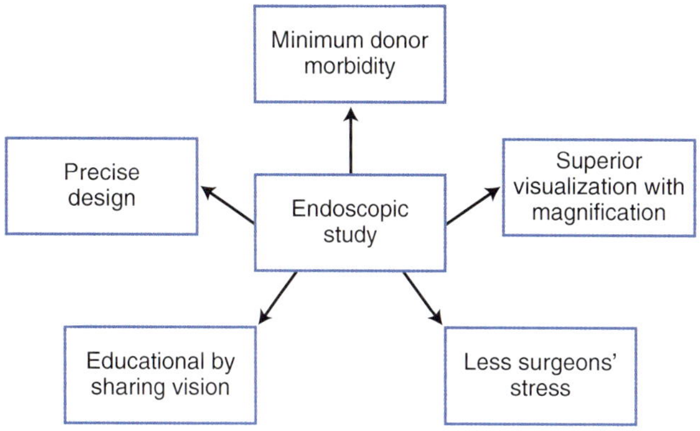

Fig. 12.22 Advantages of using the endoscopic approach

12.4 Indications and Contraindications

A requirement for small flaps or for flaps with precise design of the location of the perforators is the indication for this method. Contraindications include a need for large flaps, which would include the perforators anyway. Obesity is not a contraindication, but the incision for the endoscope tends to be larger.

Conclusions

Intraoperative decisions based on endoscopic findings enable accurate design of the flap, which leads to minimum sacrifice of the donor site. Endoscopy is especially useful in harvesting small ALTs, or when an extra-precise design is needed. The scar is not always very small owing to the requirements of the pedicle length, but extra scars can be avoided.

Endoscopy provides high-magnification, wide-range views for both the surgeon and assistants, which enables sharing of information and education. Endoscope-assisted flap design also makes the procedure less stressful for the surgeon, who can be sure of the existence or location of the perforator before making any skin incision to harvest the flap.

References

1. Teimourian B, Kroll SS. Subcutaneous endoscopy in suction lipectomy. Plast Reconstr Surg. 1984;74:708–11.
2. Chow JC. Endoscopic release of the carpal ligament: a new technique for carpal tunnel syndrome. Arthroscopy. 1989;5:19–24.
3. Vasconez LO, Core GB, Gamboa-Bobadilla M, Guzman G, Askren C, Yamamoto Y. Endoscopic techniques in coronal brow lifting. Plast Reconstr Surg. 1994;94:788–93.
4. Isse NG. Endoscopic facial rejuvenation: endoforehead, the functional lift. Case reports. Aesthetic Plast Surg. 1994;18:21–9.
5. Dowden RV, Anain S. Endoscopic implant evaluation and capsulotomy. Plast Reconstr Surg. 1993;91:283–7.
6. Johnson GW, Christ JE. The endoscopic breast augmentation: the transumbilical insertion of saline-filled breast implants. Plast Reconstr Surg. 1993;92:801–8.
7. McCain LA, Jones G. Application of endoscopic techniques in aesthetic plastic surgery. Plast Surg Nurs. 1995;15:149–57.
8. Aly A, Avila E, Cram AE. Endoscopic plastic surgery. Surg Clin North Am. 2000;80:1373–82.
9. Saltz R, Stowers R, Smith M, Gadacz TR. Laparoscopically harvested omental free flap to cover a large soft tissue defect. Ann Surg. 1993;217:542–6.
10. Jimenez AG, St Germain P, Sirois M, Hatheway M, Lethbridge R. Free omental flap for skin-sparing breast reconstruction harvested laparoscopically. Plast Reconstr Surg. 2002;110:545–51.
11. Rosenberg MH, Sultan MR, Bessler M, Treat MR. Laparoscopic harvesting of jejunal free flaps. Ann Plast Surg. 1995;34: 250–3.
12. Gherardini G, Gürlek A, Staley CA, Ross DA, Pazmiño BP, Miller MJ. Laparoscopic harvesting of jejunal free flaps for esophageal reconstruction. Plast Reconstr Surg. 1998;102:473–7.
13. Fine NA, Orgill DP, Pribaz JJ. Early clinical experience in endoscopic-assisted muscle flap harvest. Ann Plast Surg. 1994;33: 465–9.
14. Friedlander L, Sundin J. Minimally invasive harvesting of the latissimus dorsi. Plast Reconstr Surg. 1994;94:881–4.
15. Van Buskirk ER, Rehnke RD, Montgomery RL, Eubanks S, Ferraro FJ, Levin LS. Endoscopic harvest of the latissimus dorsi muscle using the balloon dissection technique. Plast Reconstr Surg. 1997;99:899–903.
16. Karp NS, Bass LS, Kasabian AK, Eidelman Y, Hausman MR. Balloon assisted endoscopic harvest of the latissimus dorsi muscle. Plast Reconstr Surg. 1997;100:1161–7.
17. Bass LS, Karp NS, Benacquista T, Kasabian AK. Endoscopic harvest of the rectus abdominis free flap: balloon dissection in the fascial plane. Ann Plast Surg. 1995;34:274–9.
18. Sawaizumi M, Onishi K, Maruyama Y. Endoscope-assisted rectus abdominis muscle flap harvest for chest wall reconstruction: early experience. Ann Plast Surg. 1996;37:317–21.
19. Ramakrishnan V, Southern S, Hart NB, Tzafetta K. Endoscopically assisted gracilis harvest for use as a free and pedicled flap. Br J Plast Surg. 1998;51:580–3.
20. Hallock GG. Minimally invasive harvest of the gracilis muscle. Plast Reconstr Surg. 1999;104:801–5.
21. Spiegel JH, Lee C, Trabulsy PP, Coughlin RR. Endoscopic harvest of the gracilis muscle flap. Ann Plast Surg. 1998;41:384–9.
22. Chan JWH, Stewart CL, Stalder MW, St Hilaire H, McBride L, Moses MH. Endoscope-assisted versus open repair of craniosynostosis. J Craniofac Surg. 2013;24:170–4.
23. Cheong EC, Chen CT, Chen YR. Broad application of the endoscope for orbital floor reconstruction: long-term follow-up results. Plast Reconstr Surg. 2010;125:969–78.
24. Sanno T, Tahara S, Nomura T, Hashikawa K. Endoscopic endonasal reduction for blowout fracture of the medial orbital wall. Plast Reconstr Surg. 2003;112:1228–37.
25. Czerwinski M, Lee C. Traumatic arch injury: indications and an endoscopic method of repair. Facial Plast Surg. 2004;20:231–8.
26. Kimata Y, Uchiyama K, Ebihara S, Nakatsuka T, Harii K. Anatomic variations and technical problems of the anterolateral thigh flap: a report of 74 cases. Plast Reconstr Surg. 1998;102: 1517–23.
27. Katsuragi-Tomioka Y et al. Endoscope-assisted preforator flap harvest. Plast Reconstr Surg. 2012;129:597e–599e.

Index

E. Raposio (ed.), *Atlas of Endoscopic Plastic Surgery*, DOI 10.1007/978-3-319-19461-5

Printed by Printforce, the Netherlands